AF757614

The Talk Therapy Revolution

The Talk Therapy Revolution

Neuroscience, Phenomenology, and Mental Health

Peter D. Ladd

LEXINGTON BOOKS
Lanham • Boulder • New York • London

Published by Lexington Books
An imprint of The Rowman & Littlefield Publishing Group, Inc.
4501 Forbes Boulevard, Suite 200, Lanham, Maryland 20706
www.rowman.com

Unit A, Whitacre Mews, 26-34 Stannary Street, London SE11 4AB

Copyright © 2018 by The Rowman & Littlefield Publishing Group, Inc.

All rights reserved. No part of this book may be reproduced in any form or by any electronic or mechanical means, including information storage and retrieval systems, without written permission from the publisher, except by a reviewer who may quote passages in a review.

British Library Cataloguing in Publication Information Available

Library of Congress Cataloging-in-Publication Data

Names: Ladd, Peter D., author.
Title: The talk therapy revolution : neuroscience, phenomenology, and mental health / Peter D. Ladd.
Description: Lanham : Lexington Books, [2018] | Includes bibliographical references and index.
Identifiers: LCCN 2018029622 (print) | LCCN 2018031487 (ebook) | ISBN 9781498576796 (electronic) | ISBN 9781498576789 (cloth : alk. paper)
Subjects: LCSH: Mind and body therapies. | Mental illness--Diagnosis. | Mental illness--Treatment. | Psychotherapy--Practice. | Psychotherapist and patient.
Classification: LCC RC489.M53 (ebook) | LCC RC489.M53 L33 2018 (print) | DDC 616.89/14--dc23
LC record available at https://lccn.loc.gov/2018029622

This is dedicated to Viktor, Carl, Dorian, and Kyle.

Table of Contents

Preface

The time has come for a talk therapy revolution in mental health. This is based on my perception that we are losing the healing power of dialogue when counseling mental health clients. It seems quite odd to be losing this since we are communicating with each other even more readily in the twentieth-first century. However, the communication we are having is more in the form of advice, judgment, analysis, and questions than a meaningful interchange between two individuals. Even communication emanating from technology, such as the Internet's social media platforms of Facebook and Twitter, inform yet may not reach us at a level of humanity that only face-to-face dialogue can provide. Regarding talk therapy, the present position suggests domination by a medical model that lacks direction in how to interact with client/patient experiences and combine them with their expertise—eliminating dialogue as a considerable portion of the healing process.

Within a medical model, clients/patients meet with talk therapists who diagnose them ("You have ADHD."), ask questions ("Have you taken your meds?"), give advice ("You should reconsider your behavior."), tell them what to do ("We are going to try cognitive behavioral therapy."), and monitor their success ("I see improvement in your attitude."), but there is little investment in meaningful dialogue that can dramatically change the ultimate outcome. It seems to be a field that increasingly wants to talk "at" or "pass" clients/patients instead of talking "to" them.

This is not to say we have not learned extensive information about human behavior, personal feelings, or neurological interactions through the practice of a medical model. These advancements show us a window into ourselves that was not present in the recent past. However, gathering information and knowing how to share it in a dialogue with client/patients has taken a secondary role in such areas as psychopharmacology, psychological techniques, diagnosis, and other forms of assessment.

This book is about recognizing the healing power of dialogue in talk therapy. I believe that the dialogue between client/patient and therapist holds as equal importance as, for example, psychotropic drugs or numerous counseling techniques. Effective dialogue is the essential ingredient that makes practices in talk therapy more than information based on professional expertise. Meaningful dialogue combines the experiences of the client and the skills of the therapist in unique ways. According to Martin Buber (2014), genuine dialogue has three voices—yours, mine, and the dialogue itself. In talk therapy, the dialogue itself has its own influential power in the healing process, a concept completely abandoned by a strictly medical model of talk therapy.

Deep and meaningful dialogue in talk therapy has its own unique life force that adds another dimension to healing. In this book, it is demonstrated by researching neuroscience and personal experience—making talk therapy more than an art or a science. Dialogue helps bring client and counselor to a higher level of healing as they pursue mental health recovery. It has its own healing properties that transcend traditional counseling techniques. It allows clients and professionals to develop something unrivaled regarding healing. This is something that is needed if mental health recovery is to find full meaning in a client's life. It instills confidence, motivation, and resilience into a client's/patient's personal narrative of their experiences.

While dialogue is often confused with other forms of discourse, it belongs in a distinctive category of its own. Unlike debate, it doesn't involve arguing for a point of view, defending a set of assumptions, or critiquing the positions of others. Unlike negotiation or consensus building, it's not a method of reaching an agreement or arriving at decisions. Moreover, unlike discussion, it can only emerge when participants trust and respect each other, suspend their judgments, and listen deeply to all points of view. The purpose is not so much to solve a problem or resolve an issue as to explore the most promising avenues for action (London 2018).

This form of dialogue-centered talk therapy challenges the medical model form of therapy, and it can be seen in the following chapters where what is presented are those capabilities that are needed to produce *avenues of action* that support psychological healing. Insight, intuitive decision-making, attunement, empathy, momentum, selfless acts, and hope are just a few of what is covered in the following pages. The purpose is to raise dialogue to the same level of importance as medical model-oriented psychotropic drugs or mental health counseling techniques when working and talking with mental health patients or clients.

We live in a current mental health culture that has accumulated vast amounts of information. Yet when therapists talk about it with their client/

patients through a culture dominated by a medical model, some may have difficulty in allowing meaningful dialogue between expert and layperson to take place. It is time for a talk therapy revolution that takes on the current mental health culture in positive ways. One that gives equal value to human interaction and experience along with medical advancements.

Acknowledgments

I would like to thank the clients from different mental health clinics who inspired the case studies in this book. I changed specific names and locations in each study to protect the anonymity of those willing to help. However, it also is important to note that practicing phenomenology was evident with those therapists and counselors who understood the importance of human experience.

I would like to thank those institutions for their belief in another method of practicing talk therapy and how it can improve the practice of mental health beyond a medical model. In this regard, I want to acknowledge Linda Zerbe, vice president of student affairs at DeSales University, and Wendy Krisak for their holistic approach to counseling students. Their understanding at the university level could act as a model for counseling centers looking for a more phenomenological approach.

Acknowledgments go out to Tish Jepsen, Penn State University, Berks, for her tireless effort and commitment to students and their futures. Her understanding of the whole person experience is responsible for student success when leaving the university by looking at the world from a more phenomenological perspective.

Kyle E. Blanchfield, a coordinator of the Educational Leadership Program at St. Lawrence University, took the time to edit this book and had helped in other projects as an editor and co-author. She demonstrates leadership from a phenomenological point of view leading to higher levels of critical thinking for leadership students. I would also like to thank her tireless effort in promoting diversity and social justice from a fair phenomenological perspective.

Special thanks go out to my friend and colleague Mike Elberty, a phenomenologist extraordinaire who comes from a family of critical thinkers, especially his father, Bill Elberty, who guided me in my youth as a mentor and colleague. The dialogue between us continues now that I find myself in the role that Bill played in my personal development. Such history deserves recognition, and both Bill and Mike need to be recognized for some of the ideas found in this manuscript.

Acknowledgments go out to; River Hospital, Canton-Potsdam Hospital, the Counseling Centers of Northern New York, Clarkson University Counseling Center, St. Lawrence University Counseling Center, the SUNY Canton Counseling Center, Hospice of St. Lawrence County, the St. Lawrence Psychiatric Center, and the Holistic Health and Wellness Program for their practice and belief in therapy beyond a medical model.

James T. Hansen, Oakland University, needs to be given a big thank you for his support at the beginning of this project where he helped in clarifying some of the terms included in this book. Structurally, I have not met anyone finer in describing the culture of the phenomenological/humanistic movement. He also helped solidify my thoughts in more human terms and directed me away from more esoteric explanations.

I would like to thank the graduate students in the Mental Health Counseling Program at St. Lawrence University for their dedication to a different point of view while learning and practicing mental health counseling. Thank you goes out to Sarah Zachary Grant for her help on this project, specifically in helping me develop the glossary at the end of the book.

Finally, to my mentors, Viktor Frankl and Carl Rogers, who turned out to be two of the most down-to-earth people that I have experienced. They were all about the dialogue, whether academically or just sitting around at the end of the day and enjoying each other's company. I am still amazed how certain people make up one's identity just by the good fortune of having an opportunity to experience them.

Introduction

There was a time when writing a book on phenomenology seemed a laudable enterprise for those who studied the works of Maurice Merleau-Ponty, Martin Heidegger, Edmund Husserl, and Amedeo Giorgi, but, for me, such study ultimately ended up in the practice of talk therapy. What these philosophers gave me was a sense of purpose and intentionality to practice communication with people who were looking for an understanding of their life experiences. Equally laudable were more existential and humanistic authors, such as Viktor Frankl, Carl Rogers, Rollo May, and Abraham Maslow, who created the groundwork for professionals, such as myself, to look at human beings in a less reductionist manner.

However, in the field of mental health, times have changed to a more empirical medical model, notably in the field of psychiatry and psychology. The combination of the medicalization of the *Diagnostic and Statistical Manual of Mental Disorders (DSM-5)* (2013) and the introduction of many psychotropic drugs to mental health practice began to take on the semblance of a common medical practice both in how we perceived mental health problems and how we practiced when treating them. The more phenomenological schools of thought still existed but were constantly being challenged by a mental illness industry that held and still holds great power. Looking at people's symptoms began to override looking at their experiences. It became apparent, at least to me, that reductionist practices began dominating the thoughts of those joining the field of talk therapy to the point where people's experiences were becoming less important—as the focus remained on a natural scientific model of what afflictions fit into the culture of mental health.

In the twenty-first century, studying only a part of a person may not fare well in the Information Age. The plethora of communication in this Age begs to understand each other as a whole person and within the differences found in each person's worldview. At a more mundane level, Facebook, Twitter, and other social media platforms have opened our senses to look for questions such as "Who are you, and what is it about you that is so interesting?" Such momentum has its impact on many facets of society, yet in mental health, the emphasis is still fixated on what is happening inside you and not how you convey yourself in the world.

This book advocates for a new wave of phenomenological thinking to change the view of current mental health culture from results out of neuroscience where human experience can be viewed both neurologically and phenomenologically. Recently, neuroscience has stirred up a renewed interest in phenomenology, or the study of human experience, where human experience causes neurological changes, and neurological changes are better understood through the study of human experience.

The following writing tries to revitalize the great humanist and phenomenological authors from the past but not by creating new theories or backing up old ones. The book is written from a phenomenological perspective where being as descriptive as possible hopefully captures some of the phenomena that seem important in the field of talk therapy. It is a book that points out the value of human experience as a more comprehensive approach to mental illness. Culture is a powerful force in any discipline, and presently, a medical model dominates mental health culture. However, culture can change, and more established ideas about human beings can be revisited.

Ultimately, it would make sense for some of us, to combine a medical-model perspective with a phenomenological perspective in forming a more comprehensive view of talk therapy. To this end, the following attempts a presentation of how this combination of methodologies would work. Before getting started, let me admit that being an expert in any given field has not been my calling, so I have tried to write a more "everyday" form of phenomenological exploration that hopefully speaks to clients and their counselors. Having said that, I am advocating for a more dialogue-centered form of therapy where the dialogue holds equal value to such items as psychotropic drugs found more in a medical model.

Phenomenology combined with neuroscience is not a topic that is often viewed in mental health literature, especially in talk therapy. However, before getting started, I would like to clarify some terms that may be questioned for their meaning. Terms such as counseling, therapy, and talk therapy will be interchangeable. They will change with the setting being presented rather than having different connotations throughout the book. The terms "client" and "patient" also are used more in the setting being presented than in making a difference in connotation.

The focus on neuroscience is an overview and does not go to a more in-depth level as one would expect from neuroscientific research. The goal is to give talk therapists an overview of neuroscientific activities as they relate to specific phenomenological experiences. Also, the term "phenomenological experiences" does not delve into the philosophical foundations of phenomenology. Some readers may see concepts from Edmund Husserl, Maurice Merleau-Ponty, and Amedeo Giorgi, but the book tried to break down different phenomena more for talk therapists to understand than for a critique by scholars in the field.

This "everyday" form of phenomenology may seem less in-depth than other phenomenological research, yet it was important to include more than phenomenology in the view of clients from a whole-person experience. The goal was to view talk therapy from a more experiential perspective while comparing it to more traditional perspectives. Also, the medical model is sometimes referred to as the psychopharmaceutical model, pharmaceutically based medical model, or the psychotropic drug therapy model. These can be given the same connotation based on traditional practices of following procedures in medicine that may include psychotropic drugs.

The writing is based on creating as many possibilities on the topics of neuroscience and phenomenology as possible and, furthermore, creating possibilities is the idea of phenomenology in talk therapy. Clients, for the most part, are more interested in possibilities for their futures than in digesting facts or, in the case of the *Diagnostic and Statistical Manual (DSM-5)*, probabilities. From a phenomenological perspective, mental health disorders are experiences that one goes through where treating the experience makes more sense than only treating the person.

THE PHARMACOLOGICAL BASED MEDICAL MODEL

This book is primarily about phenomenology and neuroscience and how it can be beneficial to counselors and therapists; however, before getting into those topics, I first want to point out two distinct ways of practicing talk therapy in today's mental health industry. For the most part, a pharmacological based medical model dominates the practices that take place in hospitals, mental health clinics, and other organizations that rely on a *Diagnostic and Statistical Manual (DSM-5)* diagnosis and psychopharmaceutical treatment. This book begins its exploration by first advocating for a more phenomenological model being recognized along with a medical model for talk therapists and counselors. The avocation becomes especially important for those therapists and counselors who are looking for a place in a model more medically based than experientially friendly. Later, the emphasis will be more on neuroscience, phenomenology, and talk therapy as a whole person experience when helping clients. For now, let us explore two different possibilities of involvement when practicing and being a talk therapist.

In mental health, neuroscience continues to have a more pharmacological input into a medical model with research into numerous explorations in biochemistry, mostly financed by pharmaceutical companies. These practices for drug research focus primarily on the belief that mental illnesses partially result from problems with the communication between neurons in the brain, especially in neurotransmission. Psychotropic drugs such as selective serotonin reuptake inhibitors (SSRI's), selective norepinephrine reuptake inhibitors (SNRI's), and many others are used to regulate neurotransmitters in the brain with the hopeful result being the reduction of symptoms for numerous psychological disorders.

The pharmacological input into a medical model promotes a correlation between the brain and the mind where changes in the brain can impact changes in the mind. In treating psychological disorders from a pharmacological perspective, neuroscience reinforces a medical model in understanding how individuals become mentally ill. Therefore, with the continued influence of psychopharmacology into the practice of a medical model, it should not be surprising that the methods used to treat people with mental disorders follow the procedures found in standard medical practice. Namely, a diagnosis is made, followed by a treatment plan, which may include psychotropic drugs and other psychological techniques, and finally an emphasis on reduction and maintenance of symptoms associated with any given diagnosis and treatment.

From a psychopharmacological perspective, this all makes sense. The brain is a treatable organism, and if we can reduce symptoms that affect the brain, then success has been achieved. Regarding other patient issues in a medical model, such as how one thinks, behaves, believes, or feels, these can be addressed in talk therapy based on the diagnosis and treatment plan that is developed early in treatment.

However, the talk therapy part of the patient's treatment plan may be determined before the talking gets started, or shortly thereafter. This is based on diagnosis and treatment putting an emphasis more on psychopharmacology and other "best practices" regarding mental disorders, than on the patient's experience with these disorders. A medical model of diagnosis and treatment does not focus on the powerful influence of human experience when dealing with mental health. As we will see later, the emphasis on psychopharmacology in practicing a medical model can miss the powerful connection between neuroscience and human experience. Neuroscience from a psychopharmacological perspective focuses on brain transmission issues but may not consider how neuroscience impacts human experience, or how human experience may impact our brains.

Moreover, let us consider a medical model diagnosis and treatment for the patient. In a pharmacologically influenced medical model, the patient has an organic problem, or at least his or her brain transmissions and subsequent behaviors are given this assessment. This gives psychiatrists a biological reason for a mental disorder. Combine this with a *DSM* that can predict statistical probability for certain symptoms emanating from a patient's behavior and you have a powerful impact on mental health culture (Hansen 2016; Barsky 2017). In the current trend, this is how a patient receives a diagnosis by adding up a checklist of symptoms with possible related psychotropic drug input and then receiving a *DSM* label.

However, for the patient, the combination of psychopharmacology and related symptoms may lead to confusion and possible mental health issues. With the use of psychotropic drugs along with physical and psychological symptoms, a patient can identify their mental illness as being much like any other physical illness with an emphasis on *you having something* without considering *you are going through something*. However, ironically, people do not say "I am cancer" or "I am stroke" when physically ill, but from a medical model practice in mental health, they may say "I am bipolar" or "I am ADHD," and our society demonstrates little effort in correcting this misconception. Unfortunately, these procedures at times can cause identity problems with patients. You cannot be a disorder even if your symptoms add up to one (Ladd 2012).

This very brief commentary, with the author's biases included, begins to describe how a psychotropic drug-influenced medical model may impact talk therapists. For example:

- Talk therapists and counselors follow a *diagnosis* based on statistical probability of symptoms that are predetermined by the *DSM* to treat any given patient.
- Talk therapists and counselors may follow a *pharmaceutically influenced treatment plan* that is designed to reduce patient symptoms.
- Talk therapists and counselors many times defer to a more medical model-style of treatment planning regarding the specific organic and behavioral outcomes found in the diagnosis, usually a combination of psychotropic drugs and related techniques.
- A specific form of talk therapy may follow where discussions with patients circle around the drugs being taken and the counseling techniques being used to remedy these problems.

If you follow a pharmaceutically driven medical model judiciously, the above statements can frequently become your experience. However, many talk therapists hopefully understand the importance of the client's human experience and realize the main interest of a medical model is symptoms reduction and symptoms maintenance. Presently, in a pharmaceutically driven medical model, the major concern is with the organic experience of the patient rather than the patient's human experience. Even when talk therapists engage clients regarding their beliefs, thoughts, feelings, and behaviors, the discussion still resides under the umbrella of a medically influenced diagnosis and treatment plan.

A PHENOMENOLOGICALLY BASED EXPERIENTIAL MODEL

In numerous respects, with a phenomenological model, the emphasis becomes reversed. In a phenomenological model, the client's *experience* is more the issue. Technically, for example, it is the client going through an attention-deficit/hyperactivity disorder (ADHD) experience demonstrated by a highly personal pattern of neuroscience, beliefs, thoughts, feelings, behaviors, and the emotional climate surrounding a person that is the problem (Ladd and Churchill 2012).

In a phenomenological model, the emphasis is more on the client's whole experience as a person than on any specific physiological or behavioral list of symptoms. A phenomenological model has a different emphasis by focusing more on the client's experiences and then finding meaning in them through dialogue between client and therapist, which is counter to hypothesizing mental illness based on organic, cognitive, or behavioral symptoms. In many respects, from a phenomenological perspective, *what is meaningful in the client's experience will help you identify the problem through this dialogue-centered form of therapy.*

The first step in a phenomenological model is not to diagnose but to facilitate a meaningful dialogue where the client can speak honestly and openly about their distress. Some may argue, "What about the insurance companies and other managed care groups demanding a diagnosis and treatment plan before talk therapists can meaningfully help a client?" A phenomenological model will not turn around or replace but can only augment the culture of mental health as it is presently practiced. Yet this is a callout to talk therapists and counselors to not completely forget the client's experience. The temptation is there to follow a strict medical model based on powerful influences such as the psychiatric dominance of the profession, managed care guidelines, mental health insurance, and psychopharmacology. Even though talk therapy may be a significant part of a patient's recovery, unfortunately for the client, it does not integrate well with a strict pharmaceutically influenced medical model. Talk therapists and counselors may find themselves going along with practices that subjugate their training and squander their expertise while losing the opportunity to find a meaningful dialogue in their unique experiences.

So again, what about diagnosis and treatment plans? Unfortunately, in our present mental health culture, many talk therapists will have to develop a diagnosis and treatment plan before meaningful dialogue with their client is formed. One of my biases in this practice is that numerous clients will present an initial problem to buffer the real problem, or they present symptoms that will label them and begin talking about symptoms connected to these labels instead of following the underlying reasons for being there in the first place. For example, telling a client that they have been diagnosed as bipolar without any understanding of what that means may have a dramatic impact on their intentions for being in therapy—both positive and negative, depending on their experience. That is why a phenomenological model usually begins with a therapist facilitating a meaningful dialogue with clients to establish a therapeutic alliance followed by a collaboration with the client—who is viewed as the unrecognized expert in this collaboration (Ladd and Churchill 2012). Beyond facilitating an alliance is the collaborative dialogue needed between client and professional to find true meaning within the problem. Collaborative dialogue is where clients and talk therapists find meaningful common ground for continued treatment. In many respects, the phenomenological experiences followed in this book are based on a *dialogue-centered model*, where the dialogue itself is a part of the therapeutic experience (Buber 2014; Ladd 2013).

This allows talk therapy to be of greater significance than following a specific diagnosis. For example, the counseling techniques in a medical model are more for counselors and therapists to connect to a predetermined treatment plan. A phenomenological model focuses on giving clients an understanding of the meaning associated with their experience. This translates into a phenomenological model of perceiving techniques in two distinct ways: 1) as instruments of meaningful integration into dialogue between client and counselor, allowing clients co-ownership of these techniques, and this allows both to find meaning in their use during the healing process; and 2) as meaningful education rather than as interventional methods for getting rid of client symptoms. (Personally, I believe that education takes place in a medical model regarding techniques with some talk therapists, but it must be emphasized using them for educational purpose is not the goal.) Techniques in a medical model are primarily used as interventions to reduce symptoms connected to a DSM diagnosis and not a part of the dialogue between client and therapist that is crucial for growth and change.

As talk therapists, somewhere in facilitating meaningful dialogue and collaborating meaningful resolutions of problems is the opportunity for education. From a phenomenological perspective, if a diagnosis and subsequent label cannot educate a client, then its value lies principally with outside mental health professionals collaborating with each other while running the mental health business. Moreover, if a treatment plan is primarily formed to back up a pharmacologically influenced medical model diagnosis, then many valuable techniques may be used inappropriately when they do not correlate well the meaningful dialogue found in the client's experiences. Many brilliant counseling and therapy techniques are channeled into this formula when they could be used in therapy, where meaningful dialogue between client and therapist has led them to using a specific technique.

I remember an intern being placed in a counseling center where the intern was told that "all we use here are psychotropic drugs and cognitive behavioral therapy because research proves them to be effective." Unfortunately, her first client presented with numerous traumas, and the diagnosis ended up being post-traumatic stress disorder (PTSD) with a treatment plan of cognitive behavioral therapy and a selective serotonin reuptake inhibitor (SSRI), Zoloft. However, later it was discovered that the meaningful trauma driving the client's pain was grieving the death of her mother. From a phenomenological model, grieving the death of a loved one harbors an untold capacity for meaning but where finding meaning in the necessary suffering connected to grief was overlooked, and an opportunity was lost for education in the grieving process.

However, with an initial diagnosis made before true meaning was found, it became possible to render a diagnosis of PTSD, since many symptoms were initially similar and where cognitive behavioral therapy and Zoloft made sense for such a diagnosis, even though it may have interfered with a meaningful journey through grief. One could say, "This is a single anecdote." Yet true accuracy in therapy may be found in the meaning clients bring to their problems (Frankl 1973). The above diagnosis may have been meaningful for the professionals in the counseling center according to their diagnosis but may have held less meaning for the patient going through grief.

To more fully clarify what I am trying to say, let me present these opinions:

- Facilitation is a major element in creating a strong relationship that develops into a meaningful dialogue. *Such a dialogue can meaningfully and creatively affect the meaning systems for both talk therapists and clients.* I believe this should be considered when coming up with a medical model diagnosis.
- Collaboration is a major element in empowering clients to talk with the counselor or therapist so *what is meaningful in the collaborative experience may more accurately help both parties identify the problem.* I believe this should be considered when coming up with a drug-influenced, medical model treatment plan.
- Education is a major element for giving awareness to client growth and change. I believe this should be an added consideration when developing goals for symptoms reduction and symptoms maintenance.
- Regarding counseling techniques, they may become more useful when being used during meaningful dialogue in therapy or to educate clients at some point when they are trying to understand the meaning connected to

> their experiences, rather than being used as interventions connected directly to client symptoms. A medical model focuses on "skill training" rather than skills that become meaningfully connected to the client. *A phenomenological model allows clients to own the techniques in a meaningful way rather than have them as a form of interventional treatment used on them, not meaningfully within them.*

When a patient is in some form of mental health crisis, it would be naïve to rule out psychotropic drugs or the lessons learned from neuroscience to help with symptoms reduction in patients. It would also be accurate to state that some patients may need these drugs for symptoms maintenance while dealing with long-lasting, chronic mental health problems. There is the possibility of brain damage in some trauma such as PTSD and other mental disorders. Psychopharmacology seems to work when patients are in crisis or with some chronic, physiological brain disturbances. What is meaningful for many of them is to find some form of stability during this crisis or in chronic mental/physical disorders (Jacob and Patel 2015). At this point in their treatment, working through a crisis *regardless of the type of treatment used* can be eminently meaningful. However, from a phenomenological model, professionals coming up with methods to intervene into human crisis should not stop at symptoms reduction. The danger is in the client developing a dependency on their mental health professional or the psychotropic drugs given by learning to cope with crisis using these methods rather than to grow from them.

So what about the rest of a client's therapy regarding growth and change? My bias is that a pharmacologically influenced medical model has persuaded some clients to passively accept coping with their distress as a form of learned helplessness and may fall into the practice of medical model professionals becoming their caretakers so they can continue to remain stable. I admit this may not be the goal for some clients or their healthcare professionals. However, it seems only fair to advocate for what is meaningful for clients in my experience, which is *either help me become stable so I can get on with my life or help me grow and change so I have a better life.* Both goals, I believe, are at the foundation of effective growth and change-oriented talk therapy. In the first chapter, we will explore both possibilities.

Chapter One

The Integrated Mind

BRIEF HISTORY

At this point, I want to start out by making an assertion. Facilitation, collaboration, and education seem like reasonable practices for talk therapists for those clients where healing has become their major concern. For others seeking stability from psychotropic drugs, a strict medical model remains the norm and is perceived as successful. The following is a comparison of two models from my personal experience.

I have in my career had the fortune in the late 1980s and early 1990s of establishing two mental health clinics on a Native American reservation. One followed a strict medical model while the other had a more phenomenological model. Both followed a *DSM* diagnosis, and both developed treatment plans. The difference was the emphasis put on diagnosis and treatment. In the medical model clinic, a psychiatric methodology was followed where most patients ended up with some type of medication and where treatment planning included counseling techniques to relieve symptoms. In the other with the phenomenological model, a *DSM* diagnosis was given but only after a therapeutic alliance was formed and the client had input into it. A treatment plan was also required but with the first two treatments being mandatory, namely developing a therapeutic alliance and collaborating on a diagnosis—let it be known the treatment plan was highly flexible and could easily be changed. Later an educational learning process was included with many contemporary therapy techniques being used.

There were times in the phenomenologically oriented clinic where psychotropic drugs were needed, but usually only when a client was in severe crisis and later when it seemed meaningful to the client, therapist, and a medical professional that finding stability was acutely important. However, for the most part, the emphasis was on meaning, making, and education. Over the past twenty-five years, I would rate the medical model clinic as moderately successful while the phenomenologically oriented clinic has been one of the highlights of my career. Empowering clients to work collaboratively on their issues seems to create meaning both in the therapist and the client. Regarding therapy techniques, my observation has been that in a medical model what is meaningful about the use of therapy techniques resides more in the therapist's expertise than in the patient's personal goals. In a phenomenological model, counseling and therapy techniques seem to assimilate more meaningfully in the client when used as a form of education.

THE PHENOMENOLOGICAL COUNSELOR OR TALK THERAPIST

We continue to learn more information about neuroscience and how counselors and therapist are beginning to use it in their practices. Twenty years ago, it would have been foreign to practitioners of talk therapy. Fundamentally, this is based on the hierarchy of control neuroscience gave psychiatry over talk therapy professionals. Psychiatrists diagnosed and prescribed drugs while talk therapists backed up the diagnosis with treatment plans that included talking to patients. The lines were clear, and the professions were separated. Counselors and therapists were in a supportive role in the healing process regarding mental illness. In case management sessions, it was usually the psychiatrist that had the authority to make final decisions when dealing with diagnosis and treatment. Regarding neuroscience, psycho-pharmacologists worked closely with psychiatry in supplying any number of psychotropic drugs for symptoms reduction in patients. The drug-influenced medical model dominated mental health professions, and it still does.

Then neurological research began to benefit talk therapists, as demonstrated in research regarding neuroplasticity and neurogenesis (Kays, Hurley, and Taber 2012). It became feasible that the practice of talking to each other raised the possibility of changing neuropathways in the brain. The door was opened for some counselors. Neuroscience was now being shared with clients and was not exclusively in the realm of a strict psychiatric practice. All the speculation about talk therapy had a new advocate, namely neuroscientists (Rossouw 2013). For some talk therapists, it seemed to give them credibility, much like psychotropic drugs did previously for psychiatrists.

An example of this credibility can be seen in such advances found in functional MRI (fMRI) technology, which exposed neural networks that are connected to specific functions in the brain and reveals specific areas of brain activity (Cacioppo, Berntson, and Nusbaum 2008). This has demonstrated that the brain can change its neurological structure and can produce entirely new neurons by having meaningful conversations with clients. These discoveries gave talk therapists an opportunity to also benefit from neuroscience, much as their psychiatric counterparts. There seems to be a growing direction in talk therapy ever since Daniel Siegel's work with mindfulness research, along with others such as Allen Ivey and associates started advocating for such practices as micro-skills training, meditation, exercise, and other brain-based practices (Solomon and Siegel 2017; Ivey 2009). Recently, these activities have continued to grow each year exponentially. Research has been conducted in neuroscience that not only benefits psychiatrists but also talk therapists.

The connection between talk therapy and neuroscience could not have been more exciting. However, for more phenomenologically oriented talk therapists it was challenging to consider the idea of becoming a "neuro-counselor" and following a strict medical model of diagnosis and treatment plans that included the use of counseling-oriented neuroscience to relieve symptoms. The questions being asked were grounded in such statements as, "What about the importance of a therapeutic alliance and finding meaning through collaborative dialogue to identify a problem or problems?" Were talk therapists going to lean toward one specific set of neurological techniques, fundamentally in a supporting role, to help psychiatrists reduce patient symptoms? Were they going to follow in the footsteps of using cognitive behavioral therapy as the "gold standard" even before clients found meaning in their problems?

I am advocating that neuroscience is an exciting and important part of where talk therapy is headed. However, based on the therapeutic model being used, it can become a very different experience for the client. From a drug-influenced medical model perspective, it holds the possibility of reducing symptoms in a mental health treatment plan. However, in a phenomenological model of talk therapy, neuroscience and neuroscientific practices can add meaning to a client's life experiences through education.

Motivation for change does not necessarily come from compliance to the wishes of a talk therapist or a psychiatrist. Motivation for change comes from within in a meaningful way when the client has found trust and acceptance in the therapeutic process. If a phenomenologically oriented counselor uses neuroscience to help client's grow and change then it should be meaningful for the client. In counseling and therapy, client growth and change are based on what is meaningful to them, not only on what is meaningful to professionals. In phenomenological talk therapy, it becomes the collaboration between the client and therapist where meaning is found. Through therapeutic education and practice of such topics as neuroscience, cognitive behavioral therapy, mindfulness, and many others, more meaning is found.

One final note on the topic of being a phenomenological counselor or talk therapist: I believe it is a myth that forming a therapeutic alliance and collaborating on such topics as neuroscience for educational purpose takes a long time. In my professional experience, it may take numerous sessions with some clients before trust is built between therapist and client. However, I believe we should *trust the process* and not rush the collaboration based on a predetermined goal (Rogers 1992). Conversely, I have experienced clients where the alliance and collaboration happened almost immediately and where education about certain topics was the motivating factor for successful therapy.

THE INTEGRATED MIND

The connection between the brain and the mind might be at the heart of neuroscience and its effectiveness in helping those pursuing mental health. In more generalized terms, from a pharmaceutically oriented medical model, the mind takes the flow of energy from the brain and attempts to organize information and energy in a successful way. One might say that mental illnesses can be organic but may also be neurotransmissions of energy and information from the brain to the mind that does not flow or organize successfully (Castrén 2005). For example, anxiety could be viewed as a neurologically unsuccessful flow of energy. Neurotransmissions from the brain and central nervous system to the mind may cause physiological and psychological symptoms for the patient.

Psychopharmacology in a medical model addresses a closed system where what happens in the brain, central nervous system, and other parts of the body will be reflected in the mind of the patient. Therefore, in this closed system, if psychotropic drugs are given, for example, to a depressed person, neurotransmissions may change in the brain, bringing relief to the patient's pain.[1] Through magnetic resonance imaging (MRI), positron-emission tomography (PET), and other devices, differences in neurotransmissions can be monitored, helping to advance a more drug-influenced, medical model perception of patients.

However, while MRI and PET scans were improving and assessing neurotransmissions in the brain, certain phenomena were discovered that opened this closed system to the outside world. Neuroscience discovered that connections to the outside world, such as insight, empathy, intuition, positive thinking, strong interpersonal connections, and especially dialogue, were also changing neurotransmissions in the brain and the body as well (Siegel 2010). Through neuroplasticity and neurogenesis research and the understanding of mirror neurons and others, it was revealed that the brain was open and flexible to interpersonal experiences. Now it became hard to understand the mind unless you also considered the embodied brain (the whole body and the brain) and how they interacted with the outside world (Siegel 2010). To a phenomenological thinker, the mind now becomes more than interactions within the brain and body. Through MRIs, PET scans, and others, neuroscientists can observe and record the connections between the embodied brain and meaningful interpersonal communication with others. For phenomenologically oriented counselors and therapists, this means their words and actions with clients count for more than backup for a medical model. The saying "trust the process" becomes as much a neurological reality as it does an experiential one.

This new understanding of an integrated mind went beyond the medical model brain/mind definition to include outside influences based primarily on interpersonal interactions between people. One of the most compelling definitions of what is called the integrated mind comes from the person who, I believe, has most effectively used this term. The neurobiological expert Daniel Siegel states:

> The mind is an emergent, self-organizing, embodied, and relational process that regulates the flow of energy and information. Mind emerges out of energy and information that flows through our interpersonal connections, our brain, and whole body (embodied brain), where this energy and information self-organizes all at once and in all directions. What emerges from this spontaneous interaction, we call the mind. All these parts create a system where experience can emerge. However, the parts of the mind are not the cause of experiences emerging. It is the interplay within this system where experiences can emerge on their own (Siegel 2016).

From an integrated mind, the concept of mental disorders begins to change. From an integration perspective, mental disorders could also be viewed as the mind along with the embodied brain having difficulty interpersonally. In other words, the mind lacks integration and emotional connection within the interplay between brain, body, organizational/informational energy, and interpersonal connections. What is expressed to the outside world is limited by this lack of integration. Painful, habitual experiences dominate over more integrated experiences. Mental disorders create a system where a person's human experiences become more limited and habitual (Ladd 2009). Based on a lack of integration in the system, this limits the interplay where new experiences can potentially emerge. These habitual experiences (mental disorders, addictions, etc.) strengthen and deepen negative neuropathways in the brain, create a pattern of disorder in the body, and reinforce negative habitual decision-making in human interaction (Ladd 2009).

One of the leaders in viewing human beings more phenomenologically was Carl Rogers. When he was asked, "What is the difference between a mentally healthy versus a mentally unhealthy person?" he replied, "A mentally unhealthy person is highly predictable but not very dependable. A healthy person is highly unpredictable but very dependable."[2] Rogers, decades before recent neuroscientific discoveries, understood that to be helpful as a talk therapist you needed to create a therapeutic climate filled with positive regard, empathy, and genuineness so that integration can take place within the mind.

It may be our role as phenomenologically oriented counselors and talk therapists to encourage the interplay within this integrated system where client experiences can emerge on their own. Case in point where a client's unpredictability through moments of experiencing deep meaning in a therapy session may be more valuable for growth and change than an understanding of their predictability through a diagnosis from the *DSM*. Furthermore, where a client's dependability in practicing and repeating meaningful life patterns through education with therapists creates more possibility for growth and change and might be a more accurate measure of mental health for some people than depending on a list of predictable symptoms. Moreover, where focusing empirically on a client's statistical predictability through the *DSM* and through psychotropic drugs may inhibit for some people a client's unpredictability, dependability, creativity, image of self, and one's ability to make meaning out of his or her life experiences. It may be that meaningful integration in the many facets of the mind is one of talk therapy's goals, going beyond symptoms reduction and system's maintenance, and where solutions to a client's problems are allowed to more accurately emerge on their own (Ladd 2017).

PHENOMENOLOGY AND HUMAN EXPERIENCE

The question then becomes, "How do we help integrate the mind so that in talk therapy solutions can more accurately emerge?" Developing mindfulness skills is one possibility since it applies so readily with the definition of an integrated mind where human experience, embodied brain, and energy and information flow can come together in an integrated fashion (Siegel 2010). There are numerous books and experienced authors that address the value of mindfulness that go beyond a strict medical model definition of mental illness. Many of this and other mindfulness beliefs have their origin in Eastern Buddhist thinking and practice and have added tremendously to the field of counseling and talk therapy (Van Gordon, Shonin, Griffiths, and Singh 2015). The use of phenomenology has its own history and traditions in the field of talk therapy, primarily from a more European perspective, and quite frankly, it does not differ that much from mindfulness (Brown 2013).

Phenomenology becomes another pathway to understanding the integrated mind, mental illness, and human experience. The term phenomenology can be defined as the study of human experience. From a counseling and talk therapy point of view, phenomenological experiences are not a psychic reality nor are they based on a cause. Phenomenological experiences have a definitive structure that reveals explicit, meaningful patterns.

For example, each of us has our unique experiences in life. However, we have in common certain phenomena or patterns that are recognizable to many different people going through these experiences. Take for example the experience of anxiety. Each person may have their unique experiences with anxiety, but most of us intuitively recognize a pattern of anxiety in ourselves and in others that is vaguely familiar. The reason we recognize anxiety in ourselves and others is that our minds have found a way to be orderly and efficient. Our experiences are perceived in "shorthand." When we have an experience in the present, we tend to understand it by intuitively remembering the essence of a previous experience. If you have a traumatic incident later in life, you again may recognize the essential structure of this pattern. The reason you recognize it is because, in your mind, it means something to you.

On a more positive note, we might call these vaguely familiar experiences meaningful patterns or essential structures that help us organize information as we go through everyday living. It would be hard to imagine us functioning effectively without the use of these stereotypical, essential structures guiding us. For example, we possess a meaningful pattern or essential structure for brushing our teeth that intuitively allows us to brush without constantly learning how to do it. Sometimes we call these essential structures "habits."

Such meaningful patterns, or habits, are also present in the field of psychology. For example, from a counseling and talk therapy point of view, phenomenology also may focus on discovering the meaning in essential patterns based on predictable habits, such as general anxiety disorder, depressive disorder, attention deficit disorder, obsessive-compulsive disorder, and so on (Ladd and Churchill 2012; Ladd 2009). Sometimes the experiences connected to these patterns cause us to have mental health problems and may hinder us from having other meaningful experiences.

Here is a phenomenological pattern representing the essential structure of anxiety that may habitually hinder us from future meaning-making in our lives.[3]

From a phenomenological perspective, finding meaning in a mental disorder such as general anxiety disorder helps the mind integrate the emergent flow of energy and information, embodied brain, and interpersonal experiences. After such a phenomenological pattern is acknowledged, understood, and applied to the client's experience, it is at this point where meaning-making can add to a sense of integration to the client's life experiences. These essential structures in phenomenological research are not used as proof to validate a statement of facts, nor are they based as a measure of probability to justify findings in the *DSM*. Their use is in creating meaningful possibil-

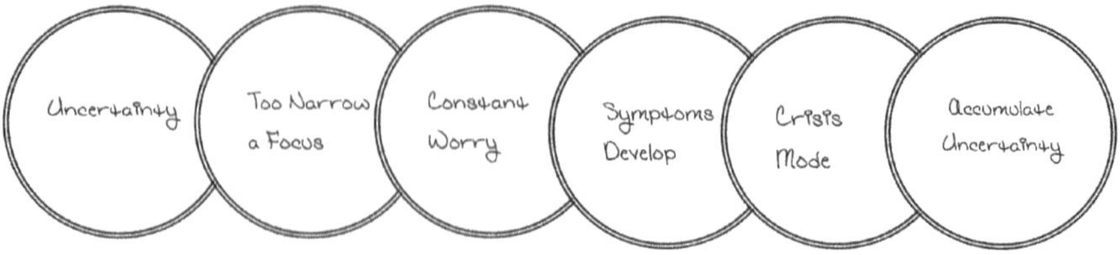

Figure 1.1. Phenomenological Pattern for Anxiety. Source: Ladd and Blanchfield 2016.

ities for growth and change for clients. These structures are based more on effectiveness than efficacy.

Phenomenological research is more about creating possibilities than solidifying facts or reducing information down to probable empirical data. Much of what is written in this book focuses more on possibilities than on more empirically validated information. However, that does not mean that phenomenological experiences are not effective. Essential structures of phenomena become effective in the meaning clients bring to these experiences.

Phenomenological research is based on a more human scientific method than a natural scientific method (Giorgi 2009). This method focuses on looking for underlying patterns that might be recognizable in a meaningful way to the client and might help empower his or her possible growth and change through talk therapy (Ladd 2009). For clients, discovering meaningful possibilities is one of the major reasons some clients seek out the experience of talk therapy.

PHENOMENOLOGY AND NEUROSCIENCE FOR COUNSELORS AND TALK THERAPISTS

I have attempted to help you with a simplified understanding of the basic premises behind phenomenology (note that an entire book could be devoted to that end), which leads us to the next section when combining neuroscience with phenomenology. From a closed system, as found in psychopharmacology research, neuroscience functions using scientific methodology, for example, psychotropic drug research to reduce anxiety or depression. However, when you begin research that focuses on the integrated mind and finding meaning in client experiences, neurological research using the scientific method is limited to the laboratory setting without some form of phenomenological thinking. For this and other reasons, neuroscience has stirred up a renewed interest in phenomenology, or the study of experience. From a phenomenological point of view, human experience may affect neurological changes, and neurological changes can be understood through studying human experience. In 2012, I made the following statement:

> Neuroscience combined with phenomenological research takes mental health diagnosis in a different direction than the *DSM* that adds up symptoms to give a diagnosis based on statistical probability. This may raise questions as to the direction of psychological diagnosis from a strictly medical model. Should psychological diagnosis rely only on a statistical probability of symptoms, leading to a diagnosis? Alternatively, should we rely on neuroscience research and combine it with phenomenological experiences in developing a more holistic perspective regarding mental disorders? (Ladd 2012)

Presently, combining neuroscience with phenomenological experiences does not appear to have the political influence, or the professional acceptance to make a dramatic shift in mental health diagnoses. However, I have decided to devote the rest of this book to that end. We are talking about the probability of changing a multibillion-dollar medical model, psychopharmacological culture. Even with the promotion of neurophenomenological talk therapy, the idea of altering a pharmaceutical-based medical model culture will require a talk therapy revolution. Such a notion requires a cultural shift where client awareness and commitment demand a cultural change in the profession of mental health (Hansen 2016). Within the next chapters, I will be making comparisons of both models to lay the groundwork for a talk therapy revolution. I do encourage the reader to join me in advocating for a more balanced model if your beliefs tend to move in that direction.

PHENOMENOLOGY, NEUROSCIENCE, AND EDUCATION

When it comes to the education of our clients, a neurophenomenological model becomes very appealing and is a distinct possibility. In the following pages, an attempt is made to show how an understanding of neuroscientific principles and phenomenological patterns can help clients grow and change in a meaningful way through education. You will be looking at the following from a neuroscientific and phenomenological perspective: making intuitive connections; regulating feelings; discovering hope, empathy, fear, insight, and selfless actions; and creating momentum, attuned communication, and mindfulness. I have found that a dialogue-centered approach to mental health allows many important techniques, such as mindfulness, dialectal behavioral therapy, cognitive behavior therapy, acceptance and commitment therapy, narrative therapy, and even psychopharmacology, to be discussed openly during client education sessions where what is shared has become meaningful and, therefore, may not disappear as quickly after the client gains stability.

Furthermore, over the years, numerous clients seeking further education found meaning in wanting to know how psychotropic drugs affect the brain. With a psychopharmacology background, I continually gave my interpretation of drug reaction, side effects, and so on. Eventually, questions came around to, "How does talk therapy affect the brain?" Invariably, I came up with statements to answer the questions, such as, "Human experience is connected to neurological changes, and neurological changes can affect human experience, and this interplay is one of many ways we find meaning in our lives." Recently, I decided to expand on that statement—based on wanting a more comprehensive answer to the same question. The focus in the following pages will be on facilitation and collaboration in phenomenologically oriented talk therapy but also on education, and specifically what can be learned from understanding the connection between neuroscience and phenomenology and how they affect the talk therapy experience.

NOTES

1. It must be noted this broad-based practice will also impact other parts of the body, commonly known as "side effects"—when realistically, they also are effects of the drugs that sometimes ends in a trade-off of one set of symptoms for another. Goldberg, J., and C. Ernst, 2012. *Managing the Side Effects of Psychotropic Medications, 1st Edition*. Washington, DC: American Psychiatric Association Publication.

2. Rogers quoting his definition of a healthy and unhealthy person took place in 1983 during a visit to his home in La Jolla, California, when collaborating with him on a chapter in the book *Freedom to Learn for the 80's*. Rogers, Carl, 1983. *Freedom to Learn for the 80's*. Princeton, NC: Merrill Publishing Company,163–83.

3. The phenomenological pattern in this chapter is based on my personal method for capturing the essential structure of any phenomena—other phenomenological thinkers have their unique methods of expressing these patterns. The patterns were developed by asking a wide-ranging number of clients about their experiences and then reducing them to an essential structure. In the example described in Figure 1.1, the result is not anxiety but a primitive map of it. Yet the essential structure is close enough to give meaning to future possibilities for both the client and counselor. These maps normally are used, if appropriate, as educational information during talk therapy. However, a bit of caution should be recognized. Most growth and change does not happen from using educational patterns but takes place in the spontaneous interactions between client and counselor. Ladd, and Peter. 2013. "Knowledge vs. Wisdom in *DSM* Diagnosis: A Person-Centered Perspective," *VISTAS Online*. Washington, DC: American Counseling Association (April 2013).

Chapter Two

Intuitive Decision-Making

NEUROLOGICAL EXPERIENCE OF INTUITION

From a layperson's point of view, intuition has been called a "hunch" or a "gut feeling." For many, the concept of intuition seems unexplainable. While some believe an internal force controls intuition, for the most part, intuition begins with a perception from some external factor, such as a certain smile or, possibly in therapy, a specific tone of voice emanating from the client. Some think of intuition as a mystical phenomenon, but hunches are formed out of our past experiences and knowledge. For example, in therapy, there seems to be a difference in knowing something about depression and knowing "your way around" depression. You can know all the symptoms that make up depression, but until you have experienced enough clients where the essential structure of depression is quickly recognizable, you may not know your way around it intuitively. The brain recounts patterns, and it is in the constant experience of the essential structures of any phenomena that helps you recognize it, without a need for analytical thinking.

Historically, intuition was viewed less scientifically; however, over the past twenty years, there is a body of anecdotal evidence, combined with solid neurological research efforts, that suggests intuition is a critical aspect of how we humans interact with our environment, and ultimately how we make many of our decisions (Lufityanto, Donkin, and Pearson 2016). Yet what is it about intuition that has us on occasions question our analytical thought processes? For example, in counseling and talk therapy, what is it that has us intuitively question a diagnosis or treatment plan?

As an example, there was a boy who came for counseling that had a medical model diagnosis of ADHD. After watching the boy, the therapist intuitively felt that something was wrong with the diagnosis, though it was the same one given by the boy's previous therapist a few months earlier. After two visits, the therapist referred him to a medical doctor where it was discovered he had a detached retina. While sitting in a therapy session, how did the therapist suddenly know that something was wrong? How did the calculated decision-making of the previous therapist miss this?

To answer this question, let us first turn to neuroscience and focus on the ventromedial prefrontal cortex's role in intuition. The ventromedial prefrontal cortex (vmPFC) can elicit the emotional responses that people deem as gut feelings or hunches (Bechara, Damasio, Damasio, and Gregory 1999). Combine this with the locus coeruleus, a minute nucleus located in the pons in the middle brain, and this combination is said to generate one's gut feelings. The reason is that the pons area supplies noradrenaline to the forebrain, which influences emotion, motivation, memory, learning, and decision-making, and because of this, it also plays a role in the experience of intuition (Demasio 2005). Most neuroscientists view intuition as condensed reasoning or swift cognition—a person's ability to exploit the brain's shortcuts (Fiora 2017).

PHENOMENOLOGY AND INTUITION

What causes the mind to make these shortcuts is a familiarity with what is being perceived in the outside world. Many phenomenological counselors who understand intuition might poetically say, "I let the experience speak to me." From a less poetic and more technical explanation, therapists might say, "I am allowing intuitive decisions to emerge on their own, based on a meaningful interpersonal connection with my client. Combined with essential or shorthand patterns in my brain and this allows my mind to respond, spontaneously. This helps to intuitively know what to say at any given moment and at any given time."

Therefore, intuition becomes of utmost importance for talk therapists. These shortcuts help the therapist intuitively make decisions during conversations in therapy. For example, intuitively being able to pick up some form of abuse in a client even though the abuse experience has not been fully revealed in therapy is just one illustration. To further make this point, according to Malcolm Gladwell (2007), decisions based on intuition fared better than resolutions that relied on rational analysis when a person knew their way around a familiar situation. He emphasizes that overthinking in such situations can lead to a wrong decision—one far away from an individual's gut feeling.

In phenomenology, this is what could be called a disciplined naïveté (Merleau-Ponty 2002). In other words, keeping one's mind open to the experience before you, only with a disciplined perception in viewing the experience for what it is and without making judgments or hypotheses. One allows the experience to emerge on its own. Let me add at this point that such a process would not be possible without some form of intuition taking place. Artists have known for years that the next stroke on the canvas does not come from a calculated decision but an intuitive one. It is in trusting one's intuition to make the next stroke count. Counselors and therapists in talk therapy may find themselves in a similar position where what is said next may need to come from the heart (intuition) rather than the head (cognition).

Such a phenomenon as intuition may become lost in a strictly pharmaceutically based medical model (Duckworth 2015). For the most part, coming up with a diagnosis and treatment plan are based on making calculated decisions where a hypothesis is made and a logical outcome is the goal based on controlling the data. In this manner, the counselor or therapist, for the most part, limits interpersonal communication to focus on the diagnosis or the treatment plan. In some respects, intuition in this model could be detrimental to the results by taking the conversation in an entirely new direction and abandoning both the diagnosis or the treatment plan.

THREE TYPES OF DECISIONS MADE IN TALK THERAPY

Let us consider intuition as it is practiced in talk therapy. There are three types of decisions being made during this process. First, consider the decisions being made by the client. If the client is chronically making decisions about their life that ultimately cause pain, one can suspect that such decisions are being habitually made (Bavol'ár and Orosová 2015). In other words, the patterns being used in the neuropathways of the brain continue to reinforce themselves negatively. Metaphorically speaking, the "pattern controls the person" rather than the person has the pattern. For example, a person enters therapy with acute anxiety and begs the therapist to help her stop the pain. From a medical model perspective, the client has anxiety within her, based on the symptoms being presented. The next step is to come up with a diagnosis and treatment plan to treat her anxiety. In other words, the anxiety is something she "has" rather than something she "is going through." From a more phenomenological perspective, the anxiety is something she is experientially going through. While going through this experience, the pattern is controlling the person based on habitually making the same decisions about anxiety. From a phenomenological point of view, it becomes more beneficial to change the pattern, not the person and help curb the client's habitual decision-making.

In a medical model, the use of pharmaceutical drug therapy combined with specific therapy techniques are the methods of choice. However, these methods are directed at reducing symptoms in a person's body and mind but are not designed to find new meaning for developing a different neurological and phenomenological pattern. Let us acknowledge that some counseling techniques do help develop a different pattern but usually there is an indirect consequence of focusing on reducing a client's symptoms. Psychotropic drugs do change neurological patterns, but they also change the biology found in the liver, kidneys, and in the digestive system.

From a phenomenological perspective, both the client and therapist may begin, over a period of time, to make more intuitive decisions based on the meaningful open dialogue taking place between them. For example, a client and counselor try numerous techniques to stop a pattern of anxiety, but none seem to hold meaning for the client. However, after the client and counselor openly start talking to each other in a meaningful way, between sessions the client suddenly makes the intuitive decision that for most of her life she has taken herself too seriously. It is at this point that the previous meaningful conversations between client and counselor may have set the stage for her to discover a solution to her problem intuitively.

A PATTERN OF HABITUAL DECISION-MAKING

Negative Thinking

Negative thinking rises to the surface as one of the major contributors in therapy for using habitual decision-making (Sharot and Dolan 2012). Clients seem to drift into this pattern for numerous reasons, but nearly all of them are perceived as negative. There are three common negative thought processes that can draw a person into negative thinking: rumination, overthinking, and self-labeling.

Negative rumination can get a client mentally stuck and keep the client going over certain thoughts without making progress. Rumination can make a client anxious as he or she keeps thinking of negative outcomes that could possibly happen. Another is overthinking. This is when clients go over and over different choices in their minds, trying to make a perfect choice. The problem with overthinking is that it is an attempt to control what is not controllable. Negative self-labeling is a process of making your negative thinking correspond with your identity. In other words, if you think negatively about yourself, then you must be a negative person. These are three out of many examples that can lead clients to habitual decision-making. It may be important for more phenomenological talk therapists to be aware of negative thoughts when talking to clients.

Constant Repetition

Constantly repeating these negative thoughts through rumination, overthinking, negative labels, and other reasons begins to form specific neuropathways in your brain (Segerstrom 2011). With constant repetition, these pathways become stronger and deeper. For example, if you put a small ball in a plastic bag filled with sand and you rock it back and forth, two things happen. First, the ball begins to follow the same track back and forth. Second, the ball goes deeper and deeper in the sand with each back-and-forth movement. A similar process happens in the brain of a client making habitual decisions. The brain looks for shortcuts, and if a client constantly repeats certain negative mental processes when a similar experience arises, it may repeatedly use that pathway. Clients may constantly repeat the same habitual decisions when similar negative life experiences arise in their lives.

Dependent Pattern Develops

With constant repetition, a dependent pattern may develop for the client both experientially and neurologically. Neurologically, a habit is forming in the brain where specific neuropathways are being used as a response to the outside world. Experientially, the client begins to perceive the world by depending on certain neuropathways to make meaning out of his or her experiences. The negative thinking combines with the constant repetition and locks in the embodied brain, the organizational mind, and human experience into a dependency that holds meaning for the client, even though that meaning inhibits an integrated mind from developing its freedom.

I had a client who was suffering from anxiety and who had been on antianxiety medicine and antidepressants, yet she still struggled with anxiety every day. During therapy, there was a time where she stated that the anxiety was gone, which ironically began to make her very anxious. My intuition directed me to show her a map of habitual decision-making. Once she understood her constant dependency on this pattern, she began to realize why she was not improving. She realized that getting better may include going through symptoms of withdrawal from her dependency. Now having put meaning to why the anxiety was returning, she broke free of a dependent pattern that was controlling her life.

Impulsive Choices

In the above example, the client had little freedom to make healthy choices in her life, based on a neurological-/phenomenological-dependent pattern of anxiety. What she was left with were impulsive choices that held her in the grips of a phenomenon that had neurological implications but also an experiential trap where she could see no way out. How many of us have experienced making impulsive choices to do the wrong thing even though we are fully aware of the consequences of such decisions? Clients have told me of the guilt they experience when the therapy we are working through is not working, even though they are fully aware of the direction to take for growth and change. My answer to this is, "Well, it may not be that easy. Your constant repetitions of negative thoughts have developed certain patterns in your life and in your brain. So making impulsive choices is the fallout from this pattern. Instead of feeling guilty, let us work on breaking through this pattern so healthy choices can be made."

Making Habitual Decisions

Negative thinking, constant repetition, dependent patterns, and impulsive choices make up the foundation for a client's habitual decision-making. Phenomenologically oriented therapists seem to find more meaning in creating possibilities for clients than in stating facts or relying solely on statistical probabilities. To watch a client constantly make the same habitual decisions about their disorder over and over again can be frustrating for both the client and counselor, especially when it is assumed that both neurological and experiential changes are possibilities in a client's life.

Calculated Decision-making

Top-Down Thinking

Top-down thinking comes from past experiences and prior knowledge that relates to new experiences. This helps us make a hypothesis about what we perceive. In mental health, much of what one finds in the medical model is based on top-down thinking (Sincero 2017). Making a diagnosis and coming up with a treatment plan is based on statistical calculations to develop a hypothesis (diagnosis) around the patient's problems. This helps the psychiatrist or psychologist come closer, from a statistical probability point of view, to what is going on with any given patient. Top-down thinking does not necessarily need the input from the patient. Based on the data that has been collected from many experts and then placed in the *DSM,* diagnoses can be made on statistical probability.

Checking for Reliability and Validity

The Diagnostic and Statistical Manual 5 (*DSM,* 2013) can make hypotheses through certain measures of reliability and validity found in statistical analysis relating to the patient's problems. Therefore, if the patient's symptoms match the statistical probability found in symptoms in the *DSM*, a hypothesis can be made about the label given. Checking for reliability and validity is an established practice in any form of scientific inquiry. Such practices must meet certain standards for a diagnosis to be reliable and valid. The *DSM* receives its scientific measure of credibility by using reliability and validity scales. Therefore, calculated decision-making has been a successful method for bringing together the mental health industry by having a basic measure for each disorder found in the *DSM*. From a natural scientific perspective, this method holds more reliability and validity than a more phenomenological method. Diagnosing mental disorders with this method is something that can be measured, rather than a more intuitive based methodology found in phenomenological research.

Seek a Logical Outcome

Top-down thinking combined with checking for reliability and validity sets the stage for medical model professionals to look for logical outcomes, not intuitive ones. The most prevalent logical outcome through a medical model comes when a patient's symptoms are reduced. This may be why psychotropic drugs have become such a large part of the mental health industry. Their main purpose is symptom reduction. For many, this is the logical outcome of a successful medical model practice. The hypothesis made is regarding a specific mental health disorder, and if we have successfully reduced the disorder's symptoms than we have logically solved the problem.

Control the Data

In logically solving the problem, the mental health professional must come up with a diagnosis and treatment plan that will successfully control the data. For example, if the diagnosis is depression and the treatment plan is antidepressant drugs and cognitive behavioral therapy, then for talk therapy, the talk therapist must focus on a dialogue that stays within the boundaries of making the treatment plan work and not drift off into intuitive decision-making. Talk therapists using a strict medical model will focus on a dialogue about whether the drugs are effective or need to be adjusted and whether the patient is successfully responding to the therapy techniques being used. Mental health professionals have a responsibility to make sure treatment is going according to the developed plan.

Calculated Decision

Calculated decisions are made through top-down thinking that can successfully control the data developed in the treatment plan, which allows mental health professionals to make calculated decisions on whether the plan is working or not. In many pharmaceutical-oriented medical models, if something is not working, this may indicate a need for a calculated decision to be made—possibly in adjusting the patient's medication or in changing the therapy technique. Many of these types of calculated decisions are made in case management sessions regarding the progress of the patient. In many respects, calculated decisions comprise the bulk of the decisions made when treating patients with a pharmaceutically based medical model.

Intuitive Decision-Making

Bottom-Up Thinking

In counseling and talk therapy, bottom-up thinking is taking the information that is told to you by the client and processing that incoming information directly without making any hypothesis, judgment, or analysis and then responding to the client. It is taking information and building on it to create a more whole experience (McRae, Misra, Prasad, Pereira, and Gross 2011). Bottom-up thinking is at the center of making intuitive decisions in counseling and therapy. This is different than top-down thinking, which has an extra step. In top-down thinking, one takes the information that is shared, you make a judgment, and then you respond. For this reason, top-down thinking appears more logical because your response to therapy is based on thinking about what was said and coming to conclusions before talking again to the client (Whitbourne 2015).

Bottom-up thinking seems more visceral, and for this reason, some mental health professionals may not trust the free-flowing answers given to clients without making conclusions about them. However, bottom-up thinking is not based on compulsive behavior but on more holistic thinking, which includes intuition. Neurologically, it is the combination of embodied brain, meaningful interpersonal communication, and an integrated mind, allowing whole statements to emerge unencumbered by judgments or analysis (Siegel 2015). In therapy, there seems to be a combination of top-down and bottom-up thinking that goes on in the interpersonal relationships with clients. However, at moments when meaning-making is taking place, it may be the bottom-up thinking of the therapist that sparks meaning in the client.

For example: A client came for counseling regarding pains in her chest every night around 7:00 p.m. She shared numerous childhood traumas surrounding her family in the hopes that sharing this information would help her relieve pain. Intuitively, the counselor asked about her uncle. She talked about him on numerous occasions but with no real clarity about his possible involvement in this trauma. Suddenly, the client said, "Oh my God, I now clearly remember that he sexually abused me in my closet when I was seven years old." After discussing the situation at length, the 7:00 p.m. pains slowly drifted away.

Mind, Brain, and Outside Experiences Connect

From a phenomenological point of view, the client experienced the integration of the mind, brain, and outside experiences, which led to the emergence of an intuitive decision. What emerged was a recollection of what happened to her when she was seven. This repressed memory came out of the intuitive exchange between client and counselor. From top-down thinking, such memories are difficult to figure out when no fact pattern is leading up to such a decision. However, the integrated mind is a remarkable phenomenon where intuition may be more accurate than calculation when certain recollection lay hidden in a client's memory. Until this point, the client kept making habitual decisions that led to chest pains each night. Somewhere in the interaction between client and counselor, a memory emerged that was not logical or cognitive. It was more inspirational when mind, embodied brain, and interpersonal interaction found integration.

Essential Pattern

In the previous example, a pattern formed around her chest pains at 7:00 p.m., explaining their origin and uncovering the experience that was causing them. From the integration taking place between the brain, mind, and human experience emerges an answer to the client's suffering. Somewhere inside of her—an intuitive decision was made to uncover this information. In a manner of speaking, the habitual pattern that kept her suffering present at 7:00 p.m. was transformed into a more integrated pattern that revealed her suffering.

It is hard to imagine such a phenomenon happening if a counselor was focusing on a treatment plan that would relieve a client's symptoms. Calculated decisions have a place in talk therapy, especially when a client and counselor's goal are on an agreed upon technique for relieving client symptoms. However, symptoms reduction may call on certain expertise in the hands of the counselor and a willingness of the client to be motivated to use these techniques. It is safe to say that symptoms reduction can take place when a meaningful commitment is also taking place. There seems to be a certain power in forming a therapeutic alliance with clients and intuitively letting information emerge from a new essential pattern of the mind.

Integrated Mind Emerges

Here are some possible reasons in an integrated mind that intuitive decisions can emerge on their own without logic or cause-and-effect processes to verify them:

- Out of the integrated mind emerges energy and information that flows through our interpersonal connections, our brain, and whole body (embodied brain), where this energy and information self-organizes all at once and in all directions.

- These parts of the integrated mind create a system where experience can emerge. However, the parts of the integrated mind are not the cause of experiences emerging. It is the interplay within this system where experiences can emerge.
- The ventromedial prefrontal cortex elicits emotional responses that combine this with the locus coeruleus, and in an integrated mind, it helps generate information to emerge on its own.
- Intuition plays a role in having new, creative, illogical, and a-causal information to emerge on its own.

Intuitive Decisions

Talk therapists in a medical model are called on to make calculated decisions to change the habitual decisions made by patients. According to the treatment plan, they decide on what will help reduce symptoms for this patient—usually a combination of talking to them and using techniques to reduce symptoms. If meaning is found in this method for the therapist and patient, the result may be a reduction in symptoms so that the patient can get on with his or her life.

Talk therapists in a phenomenological model rely more on the meaning-making that comes out of true dialogue where connections are made interpersonally but also neurologically. Under these conditions, the therapist helps the client come to the point of integration where information can flow through interpersonal connections, our brain, and whole body (embodied brain) so that energy and information self-organizes all at once and in all directions (Siegel 2015). The result is that the client and the therapist create intuitive decisions that promote growth and change. As one phenomenological therapist said to her client, "I do not want you only to get better. I want you also to stay better." It may be that more intuitive decision-making goes beyond a medical model's neurological, behavioral, or cognitive changes in the patient and allows neurological, behavioral, and cognitive changes to take place but with an emphasis on changes in a client's beliefs and identity. Such changes may lead to more long-lasting change. It becomes difficult to sustain long-lasting change when only relying on a client's behaviors and thoughts, unless the client's belief system and identity have also made a change.

DISCUSSION

In the spontaneity of a phenomenological model, education may or may not be relevant at those moments of intuitive decision-making. However, sometimes education can spark an intuitive decision in a client. From a talk therapy point of view, the concept of being a teacher rather than a caretaker for clients/patients seems a more laudable way to spend time in treating client suffering. In my career as a supervisor of a mental health clinic, the emphasis on education seemed to empower clients to grow and change. Understanding an essential structure of phenomena causing suffering imparts knowledge to clients and helps them move beyond needing a caretaker to monitor their disorders. Even those taking psychotropic drugs seem to approach drugs differently when they understand the role of drugs in the overall picture of their recovery.

As an educator, it has been rewarding to demonstrate that a client's goals can go beyond upholding a mental health treatment plan. Empowering clients through education is information that can be shared not only with clients but also with the public. A phenomenological research method relies heavily on reports from former clients for gathering information to form an essential structure of any given phenomenon. It seems only fair to share this information with clients presently in counseling or therapy. Intuition can be complicated, and there is much research on the subject that is not contained in this chapter. Hopefully, the essential structure of habitual, calculated, and intuitive decision-making will create possibilities that make intuition less complicated.

An understanding of the essential structure of intuition both phenomenologically and neurologically seems to connect natural science with a more human science. Both have their place in the mental health profession, and both can help educate clients so that they can grow and change. These "gut feelings" and these "hunches" may hold a role in helping people relieve their suffering. The dominant pharmaceutically based medical model may need to be challenged both therapeutically and politically to finding a more transparent way of incorporating intuitive experiences into its culture. Realizing how difficult it becomes to make a cultural change, it is hoped this brief understanding of intuition will resonate culturally with both talk therapists and psychiatrists—not to supplant a medical model but to incorporate a phenomenon that has an impact on so many people.

Chapter Three

Attuned Connections

NEUROLOGICAL EXPERIENCE OF ATTUNEMENT

In a phenomenological model of counseling and therapy, attunement is an essential component both neurologically and phenomenologically. Let us first focus neurologically on this incredible process. As talk therapists, when we interact with clients, mirror neurons are activated in our brains by reading a client's body language, gestures, posture, and tone of voice. These experiences create emotional meaning in the counselor and client. Neurologically, it is mirror neurons that are responsible for this activity. Neuroscientists have stated that they are the only brain cells we know of that seem specialized in coding the actions of other people and also our own actions (Iacobini 2009). They become the essential brain cells for any social interactions. Without them, we would likely be unenlightened to the actions, intentions, and emotions of other people. The way mirror neurons work is by providing an inner imitation of the actions of others, which in turn leads us to "simulate" the intentions and emotions associated with those actions (Iacoboni 2009). For example, when a counselor sees a client presenting with depressive gestures, the counselor's neural activity will evoke signs of depression from the client's face, their tone of voice, and other gestures acknowledging the depressive experience of the client. The counselor does not need to make any inference about what the client is feeling. The counselor experiences immediately and effortlessly what the client is going through.

These firings from the client's brain to the counselor's brain helps both comprehend and bridge the gap from what is going on from one mind to the other. In the brain, the pathway that makes all this happen starts with the insula portion of the brain, which is responsible for self-awareness and subjective emotions (Craig 2009). At this point, the phenomenon called the "emotional moment" allows the body and mind of both client and counselor to be subjectively aware of their present moments in counseling (Craig 2009). These firings also become connected to what is happening in the client and counselor's bodies that will go through the emotional processing center of the limbic system that will send signals to the prefrontal cortex for an emotional act to take place (Berlucchi and Aglioti 1997). In therapy, when true dialogue is ongoing, this neurological process ends up with the counselor knowing what the client is feeling and the client having a similar reaction to the feelings of the counselor (Bozarth 2009). The result is the expression of empathy where the client intuitively knows that the counselor is attuned to what he or she is feeling.

These emotionally filled kinesthetic experiences are where both client and counselor are connected in a certain rhythm, a connectedness that affects both brains leading to the transferring of energy through the mind in the form of healthy, healing, and integrated dialogue. Unlike counselors practicing in a strict pharmaceutically oriented medical model, there may be little dialogue happening. One does not need a notepad when attunement through the connection of mirror neurons is taking place. There becomes no need to fact-find how progress is coming in accomplishing the treatment plan.

For example, a highly successful counseling session took place with the client being interviewed after the end of the session. When asked why it was successful, the client said, "She wanted to get to know me. She did not take notes to analyze me. Much of the time was in small talk about basically what I found interesting. I cannot explain it, but I felt connected to her, as though she was not interested as much in what was wrong with me but in valuing me as a person." The counselor said, "It is never in counseling that the fixed are helping the broken. We are all broken in some way. How do you get through life without the experience of feeling broken? It is the broken helping the broken." The client said, "Those images resonated in my mind and made me feel comfortable, and I want to see her again."

It may be that one of the goals for phenomenologically oriented counselors is connecting with clients in this neurological/phenomenological manner. The hope is that such a deep connection or attunement eventually triggers a therapeutic alliance. It seems amazing to me how closely aligned are neurologically generated emotional moments and the eventual deep connection developed between both parties. Attuned communication through intimate dialogue and through mirror neurons helps create this alliance. It is reassuring to know that neurological elements and highly attuned conversation can lead to a therapeutic alliance and provide beginning moments of healing. Starting with mirror neurons, this process hopefully will lead to such phenomenological experiences as trust, comfort, safety, courage, and unencumbered future conversations.

Remarkably, the therapeutic alliance also may lead to revealing psychological problems based on intuitive decisions being made between client and counselor. Without a therapeutic alliance, counseling techniques, and even drug therapy, may initiate a more passive role within the heart and mind of the client. Instead of following a treatment plan created by professionals, intimate dialogue activates the client to allow treatment to emerge on its own, and with the help and direction of the counselor, a unique collaboration takes place.

In many respects, a therapeutic alliance depends on an attuned form of dialogue to emotionally join client and counselor during therapy. In a strict medical model, practicing an attuned form of dialogue to form a therapeutic alliance is not usually a part of any given treatment plan. I have observed on numerous occasions where professionals give "lip service" to this process and then go ahead and focus on a treatment plan based on analyzing the problem for symptoms reduction. In my opinion, from a phenomenological talk therapy perspective, attuned dialogue to form a therapeutic alliance should become a major part of any treatment plan. Not all treatment needs to be decided beforehand or without valuing the attuned communication between client and counselor.[1]

For example, the male counselor and female client were working hard at dealing with a sexual abuse issue that happened early in the client's life. Apparently, an uncle had sexually molested the client, and remnants of this episode were still plaguing the client many years later, especially when she was under stress. The rapport between them was friendly and supportive, yet the counselor was struggling with the conversation—she remained primarily informational with little connection between herself and the counselor. Finally, after a few visits, the counselors asked, "Would you like to see a woman counselor?" The connection between them on this subject was immediately felt. The client made apologies by saying, "Yes, and I really like working with you, but it is not about you. However, you remind me of my uncle." The counselor responded, "Look, I understand. Our progress was going along just fine, but something was in the way of the two of us connecting. I will gladly get a woman counselor for you to see."

PHENOMENOLOGY AND ATTUNEMENT

The previous example describes a phenomenological experience where both the client and counselor had the best of intentions but were not connecting at a fundamental level of human interaction. We can assume that the mirror neurons between the two were not deeply in sync neurologically, making it difficult to form a therapeutic alliance. Even though what was shared between the two was informative and productive, the inner connection, which can be described as attunement, was missing. If we look at this carefully, it may bring up the question regarding a pharmaceutical medical model's role in talk therapy. Can the talk therapist, armed with effective techniques and skills, be right and wrong at the same time? Can the treatment plan be accurate regarding what the client needs to hear and do during talk therapy but with a lack of attunement the ability to support the client's growth and change becomes diminished? As much as intuition helps counselors and therapists make inspirational decisions, an attuned dialogue helps them make important emotional connections.

Attunement is like a glue that bonds the counselor and client together in an intimate partnership where healing can begin. In my personal experience in educating graduate-level mental health counselors over many years, one distinct phenomenon seems to separate a new counselor from an experienced counselor. Experienced counselors know when to refer a client to someone else. New counselors, as a rule, do not want to refer, if for nothing else than in getting more experience. My belief is that such a phenomenon is created by experienced counselors grasping the importance of an attuned dialogue taking place. If you are not connecting at a deeper level, then it may be time to refer.

Unfortunately, there are those graduate counseling programs that spend their time talking about empathy, therapeutic alliances, and so forth, but in the end, during internships, they fall back into practicing only a medical model. This, in a sense, negates the foundation of their commitment to empowering clients. Some programs seem obsessed with techniques and procedures while not understanding the neurological or phenomenological importance of an attuned dialogue.

In some programs, it appears that being invested in a diagnosis and treatment plan overrides attunement with clients. However, before being criticized for my personal lack of attunement to my colleagues, let me reiterate how powerful a medical model dictates behavior with talk therapists. A preset diagnosis and treatment plan may become the designated activity for talk therapists rather than staying connected to the patient and following the conversation wherever it may go. Based on a medical model culture, and backed by a billion-dollar industry of pharmaceutical and psychiatric needs in establishing mental illness, all this may overshadow letting patients talk about what they want to talk about.

THE THERAPEUTIC ALLIANCE IN TALK THERAPY

In a more practical sense, let us now demonstrate how attunement takes place in forming a therapeutic alliance between client and counselor. One of the most important aspects of forming this alliance is the ability to be "present in the moment" and knowing where the client is "at" for most of the time while in therapy. The idea of being connected or connectedness becomes a major expression of attunement to the point that if you are not connected emotionally, cognitively, and, to a certain degree, existentially, a therapeutic alliance has difficulty forming. Emotionally, mirror neurons in the brain team up with the counselor's willingness to empathically listen, which helps in this connection. Cognitively, it becomes the counselor's ability to not focus on a literal translation of what the client is saying but to be connected by the meaning behind what is being said. Existentially, it becomes the counselor's courage to enter the world of the client by putting aside one's personal reality and viewing a world where a client's story of their pain becomes a reality in the counselor's present feelings.

For example, a woman in a wheelchair came into the counselor's office being pushed by a teenage son and accompanied by a teenage daughter. She was very thin and pale but with a determination in her eyes that immediately caught the attention of the counselor. She said, "These are my two children, and soon I will die, and I want to make sure that they have someone to talk to after I am gone." Her son and daughter began to cry while she remained determined by looking directly into the eyes of the counselor. Without hesitation, the counselor said, "Let us set up plans to make sure that happens."

Later in the month, a call came to the clinic, and the woman was asking for the counselor to be there at her death. As the counselor looked in the eyes of the woman who was gasping for air in a bed set up in the living room, the counselor simply said, "I am here." With a smile on her face, she let go of life and passed away. A few weeks later, the counselor found herself sitting with the children, knowing a connection was evident between their mother, the two children, and the counselor. An alliance was also evident as they worked through their grief and the sadness that accompanied it.

This story dramatically depicts a therapeutic alliance in the making. There was no diagnosis or treatment plan but simply focusing on one's efforts to connect emotionally, cognitively, and existentially with other people. The alliance may have formed for these reasons:

- Emotionally, the woman's pain was deeply felt by the counselor, even though few words were spoken.
- Cognitively, there was an understanding that went deeper than information. It was an understanding that emphasized the emotional moment that stated, "I understand and will take care of this."
- Existentially, it was the courage of the woman that connected with instilling courage in the counselor to do the right thing, to follow through, and, in the end, to be there when called upon.

Without such a therapeutic alliance being formed, the woman's death may not have had the same meaning for the counselor, regardless of the compassion felt in this tragic situation. The counselor's plan was not only to be there during this sad encounter but also to be a part of it. The alliance formed between the dying woman and the counselor spilled over when meeting the children after her death. The children trusted the counselor, felt comforted by her words, and felt safe in her presence. Such alliances can be reproductive and may extend beyond a counseling session. Such attunement encourages clients to try attuning with others outside of therapy. In this regard, attunement between counselor and client can enter any social system where others communicating with the client begins to connect at a deeper level by offering emotional support.

The connection between client and counselor may need more than an emotional response to a client's pain. It may need more than understanding procedures and techniques to relieve pain. Moreover, it may need more than remaining an observer in the process. To form a therapeutic alliance with a client sometimes may need the courage to enter their world knowing that some of the pain will follow you upon your return. In a strict medical model, these characteristics may take a secondary or an unknown role in the therapy process.

Fortunately, talk therapists may have the training to practice these skills but not necessarily "because of"—but possibly "in spite of"—medical model procedures. How important is the process of attunement in forming a therapeutic alliance for a talk therapist? Along with intuitive decision-making, it stands out as a fundamental process for a client's growth and change.

ACCOUNTABILITY AND ABILITY

Before diving into a phenomenological pattern depicting a therapeutic alliance, let me clarify observations over the years regarding certain phenomena in mental health practice for talk therapists. Talk therapists need to be accountable to the institution where they practice their expertise. For example, in a medical model practice, counselors may gather a client's history and take down information in the form of progress notes describing the experience from each visit. There also might be communication with clients regarding how they are progressing with their treatment plans—not to mention case-management meetings and periodic assessments. These and other activities are required to be accountable for a professional operation to take place.

Such activities are important and are not being questioned, but it must be noted, when practicing procedural activities talk therapists have little opportunity to attune themselves and stay present in the lives of their clients. For example, taking a client's history and talking about information from the past puts the counselor behind the client as far as staying in the present with an interpersonal connection. Talking about progress on a client's treatment plan puts the counselor ahead of the client regarding staying in the present with interpersonal communication. These activities make the talk therapist accountable to the institution they represent and are usually mandatory activities to remain accountable and professional. However, these activities are accountability oriented and are not intimately associated with attunement, being present, or activating a deep connection between mirror neurons in the client and counselor. Their focus is to assure accountability in the credibility of the mental health system, yet they have less to do with the abilities most frequently associated with talk therapy.

From a phenomenological viewpoint, ability comes from such activities as being able to make intuitive decisions during counseling or the ability to stay attuned and in the present while creating a dialogue with a client—and many of the other issues that will be discussed in subsequent chapters in this book. In my experience, it becomes a problem when accountability is given most of the time and attention at the expense of the ability needed to be an experienced talk therapist.

Some institutions may have little understanding of the practices involved in being and becoming a talk therapist. Much of their emphasis can be on accountability regarding procedures found in a medical model, and that, of course, is understandable. In my professional practice as a supervisor of two mental health clinics, I have tried to keep a balance between accountability and ability. In the past, I have observed talk therapists who have highly legible and complete forms, progress notes, very specific psychological histories of their clients, and have stayed strictly focused on what needs to be accomplished in a treatment plan, yet they have failed miserably based on their inability to create a dialogue with their clients.

FORMING A THERAPEUTIC ALLIANCE

In understanding attunement, let us look at a therapeutic alliance.

Focusing

Many stories can depict how to form a therapeutic alliance, but one stands out as what not to do, especially when considering the phenomenon of attunement.

A new and inexperienced therapist wanted to create what he thought would be a climate of positive regard by telling the client on their first encounter how much he appreciated her seeking out counseling and the affection he felt toward her for this courageous act. Unfortunately, the client was simply checking him out and was nowhere near feeling any appreciation or affection for the therapist. That was the last time she attempted therapy with that therapist.

Regarding the concept of attunement in this example, where being in the present moment seems mandatory, the therapist's actions created a problem for the client and for him personally. Unless an immediate bond takes place in therapy, when we initially meet clients, most of us have an amount of time where we, for lack of a better term, "check each other out."

At the beginning of therapy, focusing between client and counselors is the preparatory phase for deeper levels of attunement. Sometimes in this phase, small talk is exchanged, or questions are answered, or even asking some questions all seem appropriate. It is the time we give to the therapeutic process a series of "slower moments of dialogue" where both parties have an opportunity to "be with" each other at a safe and social level of interaction. In some cases, when a client seems extremely nervous or frightened by the therapeutic process, we may extend this phase of checking each other out, especially if the therapist is attuned to the anxiety, fear, or reluctance of the client.

Other times, focusing on the client and allowing the client to focus on you starts a connection in the present, and it can help with such issues as comfort, safety, trust, and connection. The ability to know where a client is at in the development of a therapeutic alliance is important. As in the previous example, the therapist was not attuned to the client. The client was simply checking him out while he was at stages of appreciation and affection. Attunement starts by being in tune with where the client is at. If the client is checking you out, attune to that moment before making assumptions that more than focusing on each other is happening. Sometimes inexperienced therapists want to rush head-on into the client's problems, or the treatment plan calls for initiation of some form of intervention. From a phenomenological viewpoint, staying attuned and focusing at the client's level lays the groundwork for establishing a strong therapeutic alliance.

Coming Out

The process of checking each other out in talk therapy is hopefully followed by the client coming out in some way. Here are some examples of coming out:

- Oppositional defiant patterns coming out in teenagers with anger or resentment
- Depressed patterns in clients coming out with tears or deep sadness
- Anxious patterns in clients coming out with impatience or quick fixes
- Borderline and bipolar patterns in clients coming out with mood swings

- Post-traumatic stress patterns coming out in veterans with despair or confusion

These and many others mark a change in the therapeutic process for talk therapists. Neurologically, it is an opportunity for attunement of mirror neurons to connect between client and counselor at a deeper level. Sometimes the connection between both can be pleasant, sad, painful, or confrontational. No matter the response, it becomes important for the therapist to be in the present, attuned, and able to listen and respond with empathy. This is not a time for fact-finding, questions, analysis, or any action regarding techniques. Attunement *is* the appropriate action to be taken.

Sometimes in a strict pharmaceutically based medical model, such action is overlooked. Talk therapists may find themselves checking out procedures in their treatment plans rather than helping patients in coming out. For example, a client may be at a point where he or she needs to come out in some way, and the talk therapist is making a calculated decision by asking about how the medication is working. Or the talk therapist begins describing procedures connected to the treatment plan. Such calculated decisions are either behind the client's present reality with medication questions or ahead of the client's present reality with information on treatment rather than in the present and attuned to the moment. However, from a medical model point of view, such actions and procedures are relevant and necessary. From a phenomenological point of view, such actions may disrupt the potential for creating a therapeutic alliance and a present connection to the client.

Appreciation

Clients appreciate when you stay attuned to them. They know where you are at, and they know your focus is on them. The ability to stay attuned over the course of therapy can be subtly appreciated by someone who has come out and has shared their suffering and pain. At this point, clients are not looking for advice, judgments, or techniques. They are looking for a connection. Continually being attuned to clients can increase the outcome for success in developing a therapeutic alliance both neurologically and phenomenologically (Robinder, Davis, and Williams 2005). Appreciation allows a trust to build. It allows safety to be experienced. It also may allow a talk therapist to introduce a possible counseling technique or at least present one to the client. If the client has a sense of appreciation for the therapist, many actions are possible.

Here was the treatment plan for a sixteen-year-old with a diagnosis of oppositional defiant disorder (ODD) and possibly a dual diagnosis of attention deficit disorder:

- Problem-solving and skill-training for inappropriate behavior in school
- Social skill-training for getting along with peers
- Medication for the relief of anxiety and hypervigilance

When the teenager entered the counselor's office, there was all the body language of someone who did not want to be there. There was a period where the client and counselor spent time checking each other out through small talk about friends, basketball, and becoming involved with girls. After a few sessions, the client erupted with anger about having to waste time with therapy. The counselor acknowledged that he could see why the client felt that it was a waste of time. The next week the counselor challenged the client to a game of basketball by putting on his wall a small basketball net with suction cups and using rolled up magazine pages with tape to create a makeshift ball. The counselor was determined to win the game, and he did so through the entire session with the teenager.

The next week, the teenager was not so easy to beat. There was an appreciation developing between the two about honestly wanting to win each game. A few weeks later, the teenager brought his own wrapped-up ball as a sign that he was serious about winning each game. However, after the games, he shared his feelings about his life in school and how he viewed his peers and how they viewed him as a bully. In subsequent weeks, they worked on problem-solving skills and social skills to help improve the teenager's experience in school.

Without the counselor's close attunement to the client and staying with him while he was coming out, the possibilities of accomplishing the goals of the treatment plan can be markedly reduced. Appreciation is earned not through procedures in a treatment plan but through staying attuned to the client while therapeutic alliance is being formed.

Affection

Affection is an appreciation that has gone from the head to the heart. In more neurological terms, it is where a deep connection is made neurologically by the client's and counselor's attunement through the transference of mirror neurons between them. At this level of attunement, more productive work can take place between both parties. Almost anything can be said, whether joking or in a more serious tone. The affection that is formed acts as a glue to help maintain a sense of growth and change in both parties. It has been shared with me by other counselors that when seeing a client from the distant past where attunement took place, and both still have an appreciation of each other that a certain level of affection is expressed by the client to the counselor. This was followed by reporting their encounter in therapy that made all the difference.

When a talk therapist tries to fix a client through a strict pharmaceutically based medical model, such a level of attunement might not be obtained. Even when the treatment plan is successful, the chances of it remaining successful over time can be markedly diminished without the meaning found in a strong connection between client and counselor. This connection may remain alive in the healing process of the client. Having established a strong therapeutic alliance at the level of affection seems to have a longer shelf life for successful treatment than without it.

Sacrifice

There is a level found in a therapeutic alliance where attunement is met at a higher level. The practice of sacrifice for another creates a connection between one person and another at the highest level. To describe this level of a therapeutic alliance, it may be easier to address it in a non-therapeutic setting. For example, when asking veterans or other combat soldiers the question, "What is the reason for your service in war beyond country and honor?" it is the sacrifice they are willing to make for the person on either side of them to survive the conflict. This also is true of firefighters, law enforcement officers, and others who are willing to sacrifice harm for the sake of another person.

In a subtle way, a phenomenological counselor may be willing to make a similar but less noticed sacrifice to bring someone back from the brink of despair. This requires a therapeutic alliance where the attunement is so strong that it alone makes the difference regarding growth and change. For example, someone tells a counselor that he or she is contemplating death through suicide. The counselor senses a few things: 1) the client is calling out for help from someone they trust; and 2) this may require the counselor to sacrifice a part of his or her emotional self to help the client. In this case, it may take more courage than intelligence to be effective. Neurologically, it may take attunement at the highest level where success may require someone to be courageous enough to care about another's very existence.[2] However, this act of sacrifice brings up some interesting questions. In discussions with many highly competent talk therapists, the idea of sacrificing everyday while in counseling can lead to being too responsible—which may lead to being irresponsible. More realistically, on occasions, it may require a talk therapist to attune at the level of sacrifice for the sake of a client. However, this is not recommended day-to-day based on not needing that level of sacrifice in all situations. Occasionally, the decision is in the hands of the talk therapist, asking themselves "Do I have the courage to go where the client is at, knowing the dangers to my emotional self?"

DISCUSSION

Neuroscience and phenomenology show us something about emotional connections that can be lost in a treatment plan that is too structured and rigid. It certainly is easier to measure accountability when specific tasks are clear and agreed upon, such as *DSM* diagnoses, psychological assessments, and treatment plans. Most are scientifically measurable and, therefore, can be assessed for accountability. The dilemma for talk therapists is that many therapy skills are new to scientifically being measured, such as intuitive decision-making and attuned communication. However, through PET scans and MRIs, this phenomenon is changing. Neural imaging can now take images of the brain and see changes when practicing attunement (Decety 2010). It may be time for the development of a mental health culture that promotes pharmaceutically driven medical model treatment for mental health problems and combines this practice with phenomenologically based talk therapy skills.

However, the drift has moved even more toward a medicalized form of treatment in mental health with the culture of psychotropic drugs and measurable treatment plans following a similar model as in physical medicine. It may be time to empower clients and talk therapist to have an opportunity to express autonomy when practicing a more phenomenological, dialogue-centered model. In my experience of developing two different mental health clinics, one traditional and the other more phenomenological, both provided services to patients/clients. However, practicing attunement in the more phenomenological model allowed me to observe the more long-lasting results of this model, along with a significant improvement in results regarding client growth and change (Ladd and Churchill 2012). There is no question that my anecdotal information in this book uncovers my biases. However, biases from a phenomenological perspective are not based on emotionally impulsive decision-making but can be found in the intuitive decisions being made by those counselors who value connecting with clients at the highest level.

Most of these decisions come from association with clients and colleagues and what I have learned from them. It is amazing to me how much wisdom is revealed when you stay closely attuned to your clients and colleagues. In many respects, such intuitive decisions are at the base of research being viewed as a human science (Dane, Rockmann, and Pratt 2012). As human beings, it may be wise to trust the process of human emotional connection, so that natural science and human science can come together and help people in need.

NOTES

1. Attunement is increasingly becoming a lost skill in contemporary society. The use of the internet, through Twitter, Facebook, and other electronic communication, limits the face-to-face communication where mirror neurons can affect the communicators. Even a medical model form of communication may not supply the client and therapist with this vital connection. Adler, Iris. 2013. "How Our Digital Devices Are Affecting Our Personal Relationships," *WBUR* January 17, 2013. Retrieved from http://www.wbur.org/2013/01/17/digital-lives-i.

2. This may be why soldiers returning from war have difficulty beyond experiencing post-traumatic stress disorder (PTSD). They may have attuned at such a deep level with other soldiers that when returning home the lack of deeper attunement may drive them back to experience another tour of duty, or they struggle with perceptions of mediocrity in their new lifestyle. It also may be why brothers-in-arms can attune to each other for the rest of their lives. Ladd, Peter. 2009. *Emotional Addictions: A Reference Book for Addictions and Mental Health Counseling*. Lanham, MD: UPA—Rowman and Littlefield Publications, 63–82.

Chapter Four

Emotional Regulation

EMOTIONAL REGULATION: A NEUROLOGICAL EXPERIENCE

Emotional regulation is described as a person's ability to face experiences with any number of emotions that one can tolerate and where one is flexible in reacting to these emotions both spontaneously and in a more adjustable manner (Aldao 2014). When discussing the neurological experience of emotional regulation, there are three important parts to consider. The first consideration is the brain stem combined with the spinal cord that unconsciously regulates our nervous system, specifically the autonomic nervous system. The autonomic nervous system regulates our breathing, digestion, heart rate, and other body functions unconsciously without us putting any decision-making need into the process. When this system is in balance, we are relaxed, alert, engaged, and calm.

However, the second issue to consider is when something in life upsets us, as can be found in clients during talk therapy, the sympathetic branch of the autonomic nervous system is activated, and clients may become agitated, alarmed, or panicky. One of the goals of talk therapy from a neurological perspective, therefore, is to help a client's sympathetic nervous system calm down by activating the third issue, the soothing action of the parasympathetic nervous system (Young and Cashwell 2017). It is vital for clients who are agitated to return to a calmer state during counseling and therapy. Another way to say this is as talk therapists one of our responsibilities is to help clients regulate their emotions.

Here are some previous examples that may help in that process. In Chapters 2 and 3, a talk therapist's intuitive decision-making and attuned communication helped the parasympathetic nervous system of the client calm emotions in the autonomic nervous system. For example, if a client presents in therapy with severe trauma and is highly agitated, by making collaborative, intuitive decisions, the therapist can help the client feel more emotionally steady. Also, by not immediately focusing on the treatment plan, fact-finding, and other procedural issues, the client may become more in tune with the therapist. The therapist then can help the client calm down by realizing that a more balanced emotional connection is being made.

To accomplish this, a talk therapist from a neurological viewpoint must consider that the agitated client's adrenaline system is firing corticotropin, a hormone involved in stress response, from a part of the brain called the hypothalamus. This triggers a chain reaction that results in the release of another stress hormone, cortisol, from the adrenal gland while simultaneously the amygdala, or "crisis center" of the brain found in the hypothalamus portion of the middle brain, is brought into action (Grecucci and Job 2015). If the client is presenting with serious emotional upset, somehow or somewhere the amygdala of that client was set off. Along with the sympathetic nervous system, the hormone cortisol is pumped through the body. The process will happen when a client does not have enough energy backup stored in the autonomic nervous system to buffer the trauma (Damasio 2000).

Moreover, when the prefrontal cortex where logic resides is hijacked by the amygdala, hypothalamus, and sympathetic, the nervous system can put the client in fight-or-flight or even freeze mode. A client that is at this level of being overwhelmed then activates cortisol as an alarm to deal with the panic, hyperactivity, or anxiety (Bennington 2010). Neurologically, the goal for the therapist may be to get the client's autonomic nervous system in balance and return his or her prefrontal cortex's reasoning power so that a calm emotional state returns. If the therapist is successful, then the hormone oxytocin is released, and it has a calming effect on the client.

That is why some clients may say, "I do not know exactly what we talked about in therapy, but somehow I feel better." Or, "I need to come back so I can calm down." When a therapist is attuned, and in the present, this experience can help begin a reversal of cortisol and the emergence of oxytocin through the therapist's tone of voice, empathy, and basic positive regard for the client (DeAngelis 2008). It is also why fact-finding or literally focusing on the goals of the therapist may be less important than the calming action needed when clients are emotionally in trouble.

This is not to say that talk therapy is the only form of emotional regulation. Psychotropic drugs given to patients are a more passive method for regulating emotions. However, this raises concerns about strictly giving psychotropic drugs to patients, as found in countless everyday medical practices that may be ignoring the need for talk therapy. It is not in question the role these drugs play in affecting the autonomic nervous system and the brain. However, for the client, there is always the chance that he or she will find a more meaningful connection to the drug than a connection to a professional who can guide them through a crisis.

Moreover, we must also consider that calming a client from chaos is not the only problem. Sometimes clients have become historically so rigid in their methods for dealing with trauma that their meaning systems[1] or meaningful experiences and possibly their identities hinder them from calming down. For example, a client is open to psychotropic drugs and talk therapy to regulate emotions but still is cautious about this doing any good when they have had negative meaningful experiences in the past where nothing worked, or when others in the past have viewed them as an anxious person.

If a client is in crisis and can recover from the crisis in a day or week or maybe even a month, there remains a sense of flexibility in the client's ability to recover. However, what happens if it takes a year, two years, or more? Such rigidity impairs the client from gaining a sense of overall calmness and this, for the most part, comes from past experiences. So between chaos and rigidity lies the goal of emotional balance (Siegel 2010). The following is a story of a client from a neurological and phenomenological perspective making such a point.

Dorian was a client who had benefitted from the close communication with his counselor. Over numerous sessions, he began making decisions that gave his autonomic nervous system some breathing room. At the beginning of counseling, Dorian was a client who practiced perfectionism, which seemed to be a set up for the sympathetic nervous system to kick in anytime situations did not go perfectly. Through counseling, he began to understand that emotional balance was important to him, and this came about by a strong therapeutic alliance and mindfulness skills collaborated with his counselor.

However, his perfectionism caused another problem with keeping his emotions in balance. Beyond the chaos, he felt when not being perfect was his strong resistance to changing how he saw himself. Feelings of self-hatred were generated in his childhood by abusive parents who judged him when he did not achieve perfection. This seemed to have him swing from the chaos of trying to be perfect to the rigidity of not believing he could ever be perfect. Or, in a more literal sense, being able to calm down only to have what was meaningful to him (perfectionism) and a self-hatred–oriented identity sabotage his success.

Working with Dorian's counselor was a psychiatrist who observed the process taking place and determined the symptoms that Dorian was presenting matched those symptoms for cyclothymic disorder (a mild form of bipolar disorder), which was based on his back-and-forth mood swings. From the above example, you could visualize how a strict pharmaceutically based medical model would approach Dorian's problem. To accomplish emotional balance, some form of a psychotropic drug may be administered along with possibly cognitive and behavioral therapy to deal with the chaotic thoughts and behaviors. With the diagnosis being cyclothymic disorder, even though no FDA drug is approved, lithium, Seroquel, or Abilify may be the drug of choice. These choices seem acceptable treatment from a medical model. However, it appears that only the chaos portion of Dorian's problem was being addressed.

What about the meaning Dorian places in his past experiences or his rigid view of his identity? It may be this strictly medical model diagnosis, label, and treatment plan that may reinforce the rigidity found in his past meaningful experiences about not being good enough and an identity surrounding his self-hatred for not being perfect. Beyond this issue, the acceptance of the diagnostic label could be an expert's declaration of Dorian's identity that seriously affects what he is going through. It may create more rigidity in Dorian's past meaningful experiences of not being good enough and may reinforce the self-hatred found in his identity. Dorian may have to fight a different battle with perfectionism when working to relieve the chaos in his life. The potential of mitigating his chaos now faces a challenge through memories from the past and an identity that has remained inflexible over time.

Dorian could learn to cope with his diagnosis by taking drugs and practicing counseling skills while unconsciously working from long-standing experiences based on abuse and an identity that goes against therapeutic changes behaviorally, cognitively, or emotionally. It may be that talk therapy, from a more phenomenological perspective, could offer more whole-person changes in behavior, thoughts, and emotions and go farther into changing what is meaningful to him and what is affecting his identity. By forming a strong therapeutic alliance where these issues could be revealed and discussed, Dorian could begin to make changes holistically rather than changing symptoms that have thrown him out of balance emotionally.

PHENOMENOLOGY AND EMOTIONAL REGULATION

Emotional regulation is not only about reducing chaos in a client's life. It also is about the rigidity involved in recovery time. If it takes clients many years to even think about recovery, then during all that time clients remain, to a certain degree, rigid and periodically out of emotional balance. Clients are coping with their trauma but not growing or changing from it. This does not mean that the autonomic nervous system, hypothalamus, or amygdala are in chaos all the time. What it means is that the neural patterns of trauma may be dug in deeply from a client's longstanding meaningful experiences making change difficult (Lewis 2016).

From a phenomenological perspective, the client's emotions, meaningful experiences, and identity may still warrant further exploration into making sure that the client has a flexible turnaround time when future traumas are experienced. Instead of completely relying on counseling skills and psychotropic drugs to regulate the client's emotions, it may be a client's meaning systems and perceptions about his or her self that also needs to change.[2] This may be where a client growing and changing is reflected in what is meaningful, such as, "I needed to be perfect" changing to, "Being perfect is unachievable, and I am fine with that."

Regarding emotional regulation, phenomenological talk therapists are looking for growth and change in the whole person, not only in reducing symptoms causing chaotic emotions, thoughts, and behavior. On the one hand, it appears the pharmaceutical medical model has a multibillion-dollar industry devoted to emotional regulation by reducing symptoms without mentioning talk therapy in their advertisements. Many of the commercials and advertisements for depression, anxiety, and others focus on the drugs being the answer to mental problems. Pharmaceutically, the goal is to reduce these symptoms much like medical doctors dealing with physical illnesses and to treat emotional regulation as if it appeared similar to a physical disease. However, these commercials do not mention the rigidity of the person and how that affects emotional regulation. Here is a story exemplifying this issue.

Mike entered the psychiatrist's office stating that he was filled with anxiety and anger over his recent divorce. The psychiatrist focused on the chaos taking place at that moment in his life and worked on sustaining the crisis at hand. The psychiatrist prescribed that Ativan should be taken when needed to help Mike through this crisis. He also recommended that Mike should see a talk therapist to deal with his anger.

The initial visit to the medical-model talk therapist was a highly emotional event filled with anger over the shock of his wife leaving him without any forethought or communication to that end. The obvious symptom presented to the therapist was Mike's anger. The treatment plan that was introduced dealt with anger management techniques where Mike's thoughts and behaviors were the focus of the treatment. Within a few months, Mike had gotten to the point where he felt less in shock and calmer regarding this tragic event in his life. His emotions seemed regulated from the talk therapist's viewpoint.

At this point, Mike was willing to date other women, yet he found himself lacking self-confidence and having anxiety and being filled with cautious trepidation regarding the opposite sex. Over the next six months, his anxiety increased, and his anger returned, causing him to seek psychiatric help with the same psychiatrist. A more intense dose of Xanax was given until Mike calmed his emotions over a six-week period when the antidepressant Paxil could kick in. Mike has now been on Paxil for three years yet with minimal change in his view of women.

This example may be repeated numerous times with only different circumstances but with chaos being the emphasis in emotional regulation without considering Mike's battle with his rigid identity. Moreover, quite honestly, the outcome of the example would be acceptable to many clients who rely on drugs to solve their problems. However, from a phenomenological or holistic viewpoint, only half of the problem was solved. Chaos reduction without some form of flexibility being created in Mike's meaning systems regarding women and how he sees himself with them could make the treatment plan a temporary fix. Or, more importantly, a coping mechanism where Mike's meaning systems about women and his identity still resist change.

There are remedies for moments of chaos through psychotropic drug therapy when Mike becomes emotionally out of balance over meeting a woman. However, since Mike has not explored changes to past negative but meaningful experiences guiding his life, metaphorically speaking, he may constantly be waiting for the next shoe to drop. Or waiting for the next woman to betray him and leave. Instead of changing his meaning toward women and his identity when dating them, Mike relies on symptom reduction techniques to face his problem with women. Again, Mike is waiting for the next shoe to drop instead of realizing that, in the future, the next shoe could drop. If what is meaningful to him has not been altered, Mike is not ready for such an occasion if or when it may happen.

PHENOMENOLOGICAL LEVELS IN TALK THERAPY

Before getting into a phenomenological pattern of emotional regulation, I would like to take this opportunity to give my interpretation of the levels involved in phenomenological talk therapy or therapy in general. This was developed over the years to help counselors and therapists visualize levels of change when counseling. It is not that one level is more important than the others, yet it seems when having client's change their meaningful past experiences and how they view themselves, more resistance seems to take place within the client. However, when making a change from a whole-person perspective regarding meaningful experiences and identity, the results may be more long-lasting.

LEVELS OF COUNSELING

From a phenomenological perspective as a counselor or therapist, one of the goals is to help the client change as a whole person. From this point of view, it is difficult to visualize only changing the client's symptoms, though in the short term, that may be valuable. This form of talk therapy begins by trying to find the meaning in a client's life and how he or she views themselves in their world by allowing their experiences to define them, not only to the therapist but uniquely to themselves. Instead of the talk therapist looking for behavioral, cognitive, or emotional symptoms to form a treatment plan, the phenomenological talk therapist engages clients in what is meaningful to them and how they want to see themselves in creating future meaningful growth and change. They spend time getting to know their clients and what is meaningful in their world. The hope is to form a therapeutic alliance where collaboration between client and therapist, allows experiences to emerge and what these experiences mean behaviorally, cognitively, and emotionally. It is at this point where counseling techniques and possibly psychotropic medication are in a better position to work and may gain meaning for the client.

From a phenomenological perspective, the whole is bigger than the sum of its parts. Engaging the whole person humanizes the therapy process and makes the connection between client and therapist more meaningful (Fall, Holden, and Marquis 2016). What takes place is getting in touch with how the client views herself or himself that affects the whole structure of change in therapy. It assumes that to find meaning in the experiences of clients, it is important to treat the whole person, not just behavioral symptoms such as behavior, cognitions, and emotions.

Another way of saying this is that it is important in understanding the client as a whole person and then other levels of change become personal and meaningful for the client—usually after forming a therapeutic alliance. From a whole-person perspective, clients can get in touch and trust:

- First, how they see themselves (identity) being impacted by negative meaningful experiences found in their past life.
- Second, with a change in meaning regarding their past negative experiences, which may influence a change in how they feel about themselves (emotions), especially with emotional regulation and the need for calmness.
- Third, with calmness that makes it less difficult to discuss distorted thinking (cognitions).
- Fourth, with these changes in thinking, talking about behavior (behaviors) may facilitate a behavioral change.
- The results: In numerous ways, this is the exact opposite of a medical model, which starts with behavioral and cognitive symptoms to regulate emotions. A phenomenological model starts with meaningful experiences and identity issues and works the opposite way by getting in touch with who you are as a person and then finding new meanings. After establishing a new perception of identity and new meaning and counseling techniques to deal with behavior, cognitions and emotions also take on new meaning beyond only being skill training.

It is a way to empower clients to be a part of an experience that is promoting their personal growth and change rather than a counselor or therapist controlling pieces of a client's experience through reducing behavioral, cognitive, and emotional symptoms and keeping these symptoms at an acceptable level of coping.

However, it must be noted, the more a counselor helps clients with changing their meaningful experiences and identity, the stronger the client's resistance to change. It is easier to help a client change their behavior than to change their identity. That also might be why the therapeutic alliance needs to form a bond of trust. This may be partially due to some deep-rooted meaningful experiences being unconscious, and without the therapeutic alliance, they may not emerge.

In my personal experience, some clients will go along with surface-level changes while unconsciously avoiding deeper levels of change. For example, a client may go along with changing behaviors that produce anxiety, but that does not mean they have stopped consciously or unconsciously viewing themselves in a rigid way as an anxious person. Medical model approaches may lead to temporary changes when the ongoing meaning put into being an anxious person overcomes the gains made in changing symptoms. Furthermore, if they mistakenly accept their diagnosis and label as an indication of who they are now, for example, "I am now bipolar," then they may even experience an increase in emotional rigidity.

This may be why phenomenological and more humanistic therapists emphasize the importance of treating the whole person and the therapeutic alliance. The stronger the therapeutic alliance, the less threatening is the change (Bender 2005). This also may be why the psychologist Carl Rogers (1980) was correct when he stated that positive regard, empathy, and congruence were the cornerstones of a therapeutic alliance. Therefore, from a phenomenological viewpoint, one of the effective ways to facilitate change in clients is to be accepting, listen carefully to what is meaningful to them, and to work from their present identity genuinely.

So why is there such an emphasis in present-day society on changing behavior, thoughts, and emotions regarding emotional regulation (Duggan, Toste, and Heath 2013)? It may come down to the fact that these are the elements that better fit the present business model in mental health. Changing one's thoughts and behavior through counseling techniques is uniquely acceptable to managed care facilities and companies. Most popular are those techniques that have empirical data to back these methods for treating client symptoms. However, do we want mental health issues to center mostly on business?

Frankly, many of these techniques *are* effective, but they become more long-lasting when clients make them their own and find meaning in them—when identifying themselves and to others. Also, psychotropic drugs seem like an efficient way to control emotions. However, without finding the meaning behind them, the client may put more meaning into the drugs than into empowering themselves.

The following example is a more phenomenological and, I might add, in my opinion, a more successful use of psychotropic drugs. One client stated that, "I now know why I took these drugs. I was so emotionally unstable that I needed them to calm down. Now I do not need these drugs to remain emotionally stable. I have found a way to stabilize myself through mindfulness, which gives me the power to make my own decisions when emotionally feeling out of balance."

Here is a statement where psychotropic drugs found a place of meaning in the client's life but also where drug use was not the reason for the change in how the client perceived herself. She successfully found meaning in her struggle with emotional regulation in a spectrum between chaos and rigidity with the use of drugs playing an adjunct role in her recovery.

What does this statement mean regarding emotional regulation for the client? Even though the use of drugs helped the client, it would remain a portion of emotional regulation unless changes in the client's identity and meaningful experiences create flexibility for whole person change. In mental health, the present thinking continues to move toward a pharmaceutical-based medical model. My bias is this movement toward psychopharmacology begins to treat mental illness like a terminal illness where one reduces symptoms at a certain acceptable level while ignoring a client's struggle with who they are in this world and the meaningful experiences that are partially responsible for their struggle. I believe without discussing the client's meaning systems that cause emotional imbalance and without working through how the emotional imbalance effect one's identity, changing emotional imbalance through drugs may be temporary. Or, if not temporary, then a possible chronic problem where, for example, a patient needs to continue taking drugs because they believe that they have a mental illness exclusively.

The question may come down to, "How do you balance a model based on coping (pharmaceutical medical model) with a model based on healing (phenomenological model)? The medical model has proven time and again that it can stabilize chaos so that it does not turn into a crisis. The phenomenological model empowers the client to prove for themselves the ability to find meaning in emotional regulation that allows for more flexibility when regulating one's emotions.

PSYCHOPHARMACEUTICAL APPROACH

Take the example of a person entering a mental health clinic with severe anxiety and occasional panic attacks. A diagnosis is given. A treatment plan is developed, and the patient's behavior, thoughts, and emotions are addressed. A part of the treatment plan focuses on the patient's thoughts and behavior. Cognitive/behavioral therapy is described to the patient as a method for changing irrational thoughts leading to anxious or panicky behavior, along with the reasons why this technique is effective. The patient delves into those irrational thoughts that are responsible for presenting panic and anxiety, and the talk therapist continues to go deeper as to where these thoughts and behaviors are coming from. Homework is assigned at both levels.

At the present levels of thinking and behavior, the therapist guides and controls the treatment plan. Later at deeper levels of meaning in finding the root cause of these thoughts and behavior, the therapist again controls and guides the progress of the patient. The goal of this approach is to find those thoughts and behaviors that are leading to an emotional imbalance in the patient. If successful, eventually the patient will experience a sense of emotional calm and where the autonomic nervous system has returned to a calmer state.

Along with the talk therapist's treatment plan will be a psychiatric prescription for some combination of psychotropic drugs to effectively neutralize the chaos being experienced by the patient. An immediate prescription may call for an antianxiety drug to relieve the stress on the autonomic nervous system, followed by a more, long-lasting antidepressant to take over when it has eventually kicked in. Depending on the age, prior traumatic experiences, and the success of talk therapy, the person could be on the antidepressant for a minimum of twelve to eighteen months, or for a much longer time, and even for life. The hope is that the brain, body, and especially the autonomic nervous system will adjust to this drug. If the patient cannot regulate his or her emotions under this regiment, either there may be an increase in dosage or a change in antidepressant until a successful regulation takes place within the patient.

Let it be noted that the above description may not fit all psychopharmaceutical medical model practices, but for the sake of this discussion, let us assume that it stands for a basic approach to this model. Overall, it appears that relieving the chaos in the patient's life has been addressed through both talk therapy and psychotropic drugs. Furthermore, the cognitive/behavioral approach may have eventually uncovered the core beliefs of the patient, which would address some of the meaningful experiences that led to anxiety and panic and such a practice could even touch on the patient's identity. And yet, it appears that reduction in the chaos of the patient is the major goal.

However, it also makes more sense to connect rigid meaningful experiences of the patient and her or his identity through a formed therapeutic alliance where conscious and unconscious meaning can emerge on its own. Behavior, thoughts, and emotions can cause a patient chaos, but negative meaning systems based on individual, social, and cultural experiences can unconsciously dig the patient into emotional patterns that are not addressed easily when focusing on symptoms. Excellent counseling skills could be learned by the patient, and even when the patient practices these skills, without identity change or changes in individual, social, or cultural meaning in the patient's life, he or she may drift backward. Thoughts, behaviors, and emotions connected to a client's unchanged identity and meaningful experiences in life may not support effective emotional regulation. Or, another option could be to stay on psychotropic drugs as the remedy for emotional regulation, even though the patient may still see his self or herself as an anxious person with no change in meaningful experiences to refute their identity.

PHENOMENOLOGICAL APPROACH

Again, take the example of a person entering a mental health clinic with severe anxiety and occasional panic attacks. The counselor wants to stay attuned to where the client is at, and if the client speaks about severe anxiety and panic attacks, the counselor stays attuned by listening to the client's experiences. The more the client begins to come out about these experiences, the more the counselor becomes attuned to the meaning behind these experiences.

It may turn out that the client's experiences are individually based where it would mean something to the client to receive some form of immediate relief from the panic attacks through psychotropic drugs. At this point, the counselor would set up procedures for that to happen. It may be the meaning involved is more cultural where peer pressure and family pressure has added meaning to the anxiety and panic. The counselor may point out how such pressure seems to be affecting the client's identity, or it may be the meaning is more of a psycho/social nature, where the client has lost confidence in functioning successfully in everyday life. The counselor may then focus on more positive aspects of the client's life. Or, it may be an existential crisis where fear of death may haunt the client, which is affecting how the client sees himself or herself. At this point, the counselor may focus on existential fears of identity surrounding the anxiety and panic.

It could be these issues or any number of issues that have caused negative meaning in the client's life and have affected how the client views himself or herself. The role of the counselor is not to make calculated decisions regarding what the client should now do to deal with anxiety and panic. The counselor's role is to make intuitive decisions that help the client move forward in changing the meaning in their life toward growth and change and how these changes affect his or her identity as a whole person.

At this point regarding the client's thoughts and behavior, an intuitive decision may emerge to try cognitive/behavioral therapy or acceptance and commitment therapy or others that seem to hold meaning for the client. Regarding emotional regulation, it may be that it means something to the client to continue taking psychotropic drugs, or the client may believe it is more meaningful to try mindfulness techniques or exercise or any number of techniques that hold meaning for the client.

The difference between this model and a more pharmaceutical medical model is that it remains client-driven with intuitive input from the counselor that mediates a meaningful dialogue between the suffering of the client and the knowledge and expertise of the counselor. More importantly, regarding emotional regulation, the client has attempted, with the counselor's help, to not only reduce the chaos produced from anxiety and panic but also has created flexibility in past rigid meaning systems that have held the client back from meaningful growth and change based on experiencing anxiety and panic.

One point of confusion that may need clarification is the use of psychotropic drugs. Some may say an experiential model should make a statement against using them. My personal belief is that there may be a significant difference between using psychotropic drugs as a remedy to relieve symptoms for emotional regulation problems and using them as an adjunct treatment of what is meaningful to the client. After a client has changed meaning systems responsible for anxiety and panic by making aware choices, it seems emotional regulation has a more long-lasting chance of staying regulated in the client's life if what is meaningful to the client is followed—including psychotropic drugs. A phenomenological point of view advocates for diversity when it comes to client treatment where each client drives their agenda and where the agenda is meaningful to the client.

DISCUSSION

Granted, the phenomenological approach is explained more by human experience than by empirical data. More qualitative research rather than empirical evidence shows the importance of understanding meaning-making in a client's life. However, it does point out how making a hypothesis early on in a pharmaceutically driven medical model may be premature until what is meaningful to the client is uncovered by both client and counselor. In this regard, the idea of the whole person being bigger than a sum of a person's parts makes sense. Empowering clients to find their personal meaning in an experience neurologically and phenomenologically, such as emotional regulation, may give the client a sense of "I can!" regarding the personal ability to regulate emotions in the future (Lopez, Pedrotti, and Snyder 2014). It may be that creating possibilities for emotional regulation over time is as important for the whole person than experts only relieving symptoms causing deregulation in the present.

NOTES

1. James T. Hansen outlines how meaning systems shape the way we come to understand ourselves, others, and the world around us. He makes the convincing case that because these ways are the omnipresent shaping forces of life, meaning systems should be a primary consideration when attempting to alleviate psychological suffering. Hansen, James. 2016. *Meaning Systems and Mental Health Culture: Critical Perspectives on Contemporary Counseling and Psychotherapy*. Lanham, MD: Lexington Books, 1–18.
2. Hansen begins by defining meaning systems: "Meaning systems are the ways in which people structure and make sense of the world on individual, social, and cultural levels." Meaning-making is an individual process, the assumptive world we create, a social process, where the meaning-creation process happens between people and not solely within them and is highly influenced by the culture in which we live. Moreover, all meaning systems are central to the healing process. Hansen, James, 2016. *Meaning Systems and Mental Health Culture: Critical Perspectives on Contemporary Counseling and Psychotherapy*. Lanham, MD: Lexington Books, 57–93.

Chapter Five

Empathic Interactions

In a pharmaceutical medical model, clients are asked to help the therapist in numerous ways. During counseling from this model, clients are asked to answer questions, give information for analysis, and tell their problems so the counselor can make judgments and respond to advice. These activities focus on the counselor as an expert. Much of this interaction is for the counselor to focus on the diagnosis and treatment plan. In these interactions, the center of control is given over to the expert. When patients are experiencing new counseling skills, it is the expert's role as a trainer that evaluates what comes next in the lesson plan. Patients follow the lead of the counselor to direct them toward mental wellness.

In a phenomenological model of talk therapy, these interactions may also happen, yet there is one interaction that stands out over the rest. It is the interaction between client and counselor called empathy. With empathy, clients are asking the counselor to do something—listen to the client so they can find a way to be more responsible for the meaning in their lives.

I would like to use the metaphor of a literary play. Clients are both the actors and directors in the play. They must find the direction to take in making their lives meaningful, and they must act out their unique, meaningful experiences according to their own purpose and meaning in life. The counselor or therapist's role is that of a "stagehand." They set the stage for the play to start and continue. However, this humble role can have great significance in the life of clients. Most clients who live their pain 24/7 are closer to it than anyone else—maybe too close. Without someone helping to set the stage for change, their actions and directions may not be in a position to change. One of the most important interactions a phenomenologically oriented talk therapist can give to clients is to listen empathically—so that the stage can be set and the play can go on.

NEUROSCIENCE AND EMPATHY

What happens neurologically when a medical model expert asks a patient to do something such as answer questions, give information for analysis, state the problem for making a judgment, and respond to advice? In these activities, it is the expectation from the counselor that he or she needs information from the patient to back up a diagnosis, act out a treatment plan, assess how the treatment plan is working, or initiate a new counseling technique. Medical model counselors rely on this type of objective information from patients so that they can make calculated decisions to proceed in counseling successfully.

Neurologically, this type of objective information gathering involves the prefrontal cortex, which is the highest evolved part of the brain. It is the seat of our "executive function"—our ability to think objectively and consciously, plan, organize, analyze, make decisions, and comprehend complex information and relationships (Luke 2015). However, when we gather information from a patient as a medical model expert, or when a patient shares objective information with a counselor, neither may be receiving all the information they are capable of sharing during counseling. Patients and counselors may be subconsciously putting up roadblocks to receiving accurate information. When patients and counselors interact, both parties must focus and hold each other's attention to apply successful prefrontal cognition (Littrell 2015). With insufficient concentration, patient and counselor neural networks may be weak and/or incomplete and fail to form adequately to embed all that can be learned (Kumfor and Tu 2015).

This can be concerning to the medical model counselor when asking the patient to do something, for example, "Tell me about your depression." The counselor takes the information given and associates it with their prior learning, either gathered from the *DSM* or stored in the hippocampus (memory center) in the midsection of the counselor's brain. Moreover, without becoming too technical, one could state it is the prefrontal cortex and the memories from the hippocampus that help the counselor with objective interactions with patients.

If that was too confusing, here is another example. When asking for information about a patient's mental health problems, the counselor uses her or his prefrontal cortex in association with prior memories of depressed people that she or he has stored in their hippocampus. The medical model counselor then tries to match this information with the symptoms in the *DSM* regarding the patient's depression, takes this information and forms a treatment plan around it, or takes this information to a case-management session where all participants add their opinions in forming treatment. In all these cases, the objective information gathered and agreed upon will be the focus of counseling.

In contrast, a different process is used in a more phenomenologically oriented counselor when asking about a client's mental health problems. From a more phenomenological/neurological perspective, the counselor is open to the client sharing *where they are at* in the present. If the counselor is working in a medical model facility, she or he may collect information from the client much like a medical model counselor; however, the goal is to separate objective information gathering from more subjective information where the counselor is listening with empathy and staying attuned to the client's emotions in establishing a therapeutic alliance.[1]

What can be missing in a more medical model counseling practice is that emotions are integral to thinking and learning. We tend to be egocentric as human beings, especially when acting as experts, but there is a part of the brain that helps correct being self-centered and self-serving. The supramarginal gyrus is the area of the brain that helps us to differentiate our own emotional state from that of other people and is responsible for empathy and compassion. This supramarginal gyrus is a unit of the cerebral cortex and is located at the interface of the parietal, temporal, and frontal lobes (Ecker, Ticic, and Hulley 2012).

Another area that may be missing in an expert approach to clients is mirror neurons that are responsible for imitating the mood, facial expression, and, basically, the emotional state of a client, so they understand the counselor is experiencing them (Iacoboni 2006). Another missed opportunity during information gathering in a medical model approach is the lack of using the amygdala. A small almond-shaped part of our inner brain, it is the seat of emotions and elicits the emotional response component of our behavior. Amygdala activation during the encoding of information gathering between client and counselor enhances their subsequent retrieval through both getting a dopamine reward. This means that emotional cues added to information gathering forge a deeper and richer neural pathway than fact-based content alone (Lang and Bradley 2010). It is not that objective information and knowledge gathered by the counselor about the client is not important. However, much of that information and knowledge is for accountability purposes more than emotionally interacting with clients.

Furthermore, the practice of empathy does not only focus on the client supplying objective information for counselors. Empathy becomes a combination of integration between the supramarginal gyrus, hippocampus, and amygdala but also the second "brain" of the client, the gut. Empathy depends on the gut to send signals to the cerebral cortex to gather not only objective information but also subject information, especially emotional information. The brain in your head isn't your only brain. There's a "second brain" in your intestines that contains a hundred million neurons. Gut bacteria are responsible for making over thirty neurotransmitters, including serotonin (Carpenter 2012). What makes empathy so powerful in the practice of counseling is its ability to integrate the supramarginal gyrus, cerebral cortex, mirror neurons, amygdala, hippocampus, and the gut when listening and responding to clients. In a medical model, the levels of intensity in these neurological functions are diminished (Carpenter 2012).

Also, empathic information that is shared between client and counselor affects client motivation. Lack of motivation can become a barrier if the counselor takes on the objective tone of an expert or the client does not connect with the counselor's medical model fact-finding approach—and perceives no value, lacks interest, is overwhelmed, or is fearful of the information gathering of the counselor. In any of these cases, without a therapeutic alliance, there may be little intrinsic incentive to learn about each other. Under these conditions, the dopamine reward mechanisms, necessary to stimulate and reinforce learning, may fail to be activated at any significant level for either party (Daw and Tobler 2014).

Let's discuss one other note on a medical model approach to gathering information from the client. A roadblock may be in asking for too much objective information or "information overload" from the client that may reduce the quality of the information given. The amount of fact-finding that goes on in many pharmaceutically based medical models before a therapeutic alliance is formed may cause an emotional barrier between client and counselor and may be an intrinsic factor when learning about, diagnosing, and treating a client. Too much information gathering can send the signal that counseling is about helping the counselor fix the client, rather than the client finding meaning in changing his or her life experiences. Here is an actual story depicting some of the fallout from a medical model. The story emphasizes an extreme example, yet less extreme examples often happen when using a strictly pharmaceutically based medical model.

Jim entered the mental health clinic in bad shape. He was paralyzed with anxiety and needed to talk with someone about the crisis he was in. The first person he spoke with was an intake worker who had him fill out numerous forms and collected information about insurance, brief family history, former occurrences, signing of informed consent agreements, and other information needed before he met with the psychiatrist for observation. This was the beginning of the data-collection process that he would experience. When meeting with the psychiatrist, the data collection continued. Appearance, clothing, and hygiene were all recorded along with his behavior, motor activity, and eye contact. The psychiatrist was also looking at his speech and thought processes and determined his affect and mood. Much of this information was written down in front of him as the data gathering continued. The psychiatrist was looking for his ability to make judgments and insights into his problem. The psychiatrist also asked about his sleeping habits, family history of mental illness, medical illness, and substance abuse. At the end of the interview, the psychiatrist decided on the clinical significance of these observations and made an evaluation. Jim was also given a mental status exam. A prescription for Ativan and Zoloft was given, and he was scheduled to meet with a counselor to deal with his anxiety.

Using the *DSM*, the psychiatrist made the diagnosis that Jim was suffering from general anxiety disorder and depression based on the symptoms he presented, and the next week, Jim met with a counselor and began therapy. Based on the psychiatrist's observations, the counselor asked about his childhood and his relationship with his father. Jim had mentioned that he favored his mother over his father in his interview but not to the extent that any abuse occurred or that he wanted to talk about this with anyone. After going down this path for a while, Jim told the counselor that he was here to talk about his anxiety and how he was burned out from his work as a parole officer to the point where he felt paralyzed with anxiety.

The counselor then switched the conversation to his work and asked him why he was still working even though he mentioned work as a part of his problem. Jim shared that even though his work was exhausting, he still wanted to work based on it having meaning in his life. The counselor listened but found it difficult to understand how he could work in such an anxiety-ridden condition. Later in the week after the counseling session, the counselor reported what she felt was his obsession with work during a case-management meeting that added a new diagnosis to his chart: obsessive-compulsive disorder.

In the weeks that followed, the counselor tried numerous counseling techniques to deal with Jim's general anxiety disorder, such as reframing, cognitive restructuring, ration-emotive behavioral therapy, journaling, and systematic desensitization for his anxiety and obsessive-compulsive tendencies. None of these seemed to work based on Jim's complaints about feeling sick and anxious and that he felt the drugs were making him sick. In another case-management meeting with the psychiatrist and others, it was recommended that his dosage for the antidepressant should be increased and that his attitude seemed inflexible regarding work, leading to reinforcing the diagnosis of obsessive-compulsive disorder.

When Jim eventually found blood in his urine, he decided to cancel his appointments with the counselor at the mental health clinic and check in with his family medical doctor, who ran tests and decided the drug was causing problems with his kidneys. However, when his medical doctor received his file from the mental health clinic, it stated that he was noncompliant with therapy and that his leaving was based on his decision not to seek further treatment. Jim eventually pulled out of his anxiety without missing one day of work, the one activity that held significant meaning for him during this ordeal. However, what the anxiety meant to him still seemed a mystery.

PHENOMENOLOGY AND EMPATHY

There are some questions that could be asked by a phenomenology oriented mental health professional about the abovementioned story, such as where is the empathy, or where does the gut of the mental health professionals or client enter the sessions held by the mental health clinic? Is there room for subjective information to compliment objective information? From a phenomenological model, what is the purpose of making assumptions about one's appearance, clothing, hygiene, behavior, motor activity, eye contact, thought processes, affect, or mood? Why are these observations made at a distance with no empathic or emotional contact with the client to find meaning in these observations? Why was no attempt to integrate the thoughts and emotions of the mental health professionals and the client in understanding what is meaningful for continuing the process? For example, maybe Jim had trouble during information gathering in articulating his relationship with his father while under paralyzing anxiety. Maybe Jim found meaning in not stopping his work even though it may not make logical sense to continue working under those anxious conditions, and maybe Jim happens to be a sloppy dresser.

Practicing empathy in all these observations could change the direction of the mental health process. Observations made through objective information gathering appear to discount the subjective experiences of the client. For example, if the psychiatrist was not intent on gathering objective information to make a diagnosis, he may look for emotional information and noticed that Jim was paralyzed with anxiety, which meant something to him. He could have asked what all this meant and listened empathically to Jim's story. The counselor could have empathically listened to the meaning behind why Jim wanted to stay at work instead of associating work with obsessive-compulsive disorder. Regarding the protocol for Jim's regiment of drugs, it may have meant that drugs were necessary for Jim to calm down, but only in the context of calming down and not in solving his problem. Moreover, instead of changing the dosage of the drug to relieve Jim's anxious symptoms, he could have believed that Jim was getting physically ill.

Even though a medical model may ask a copious amount of information, the information still may be incomplete to help a client without an empathic, subjective dialogue between professional and client. Within a phenomenological perspective, there is a time and place for gathering accurate information, and that is while forming a therapeutic alliance between professionals and clients. Empathic listening and interactive dialogue connect both objective and subjective information from the prefrontal cortex, amygdala, mirror neurons, supramarginal gyrus, hippocampus, and gut—information that helps client and counselor accurately continue in counseling.[2]

FORMING AN OBJECTIVE INTERACTION

Patient Talks

Either when a patient talks to the counselor or the counselor talks to the patient, a chain of interaction begins where information is shared between both parties. In a pharmaceutical medical model, the immediate information that the counselor is looking for is very similar to information that is sought after by a medical doctor. There is a gathering of objective information asked by the mental health professional, whether it is by the intake person, psychiatrist, or a mental health counselor, it is a form of fact-finding where the focus is on the information and not the client. These professionals set the tone for how the client talks. If the professionals are asking objective questions, then the client most likely will be answering with more objective answers. This is usually done in a professional manner from what clients have grown to expect from experts. The client gives more objective information so that the expert can eventually make a diagnosis and formulate a treatment plan based on what is observed by the professional. What becomes most important to the professional is what is objectively observed while the patient is talking.

Relate to Observable Information

When the patient begins to interact with a medical model professional, what is said by the patient and what is observed by the professional could be called objective and observable information gathering. In many respects, this is a one-sided process where a patient talks and the professional observes while gathering objective and professional information on the patient. The main concern is for the professional to gather information, and, therefore, the focus stays mainly with the professional and what he or she finds observably important. Usually, this puts the patient in the passive role of information giver and the professional in the active role of information receiver, based on this information being used in a diagnosis and treatment plan made up by expert professionals.

Use of Objective Mind

What is then called for by these professionals, who may include a psychiatrist or counselor, is to use their objective minds to gather more information, and the objective mind relies on different interactions to receive this information. Questioning is an interaction that takes existing information and asks the patient to add to that information, or by asking probing questions, such as found in attempting to isolate mental health symptoms. Analysis takes the patient's information and tries to put it together to arrive at, for example, a diagnosis. Judgments are made when enough information is gathered, and the patient is judged as having a mental disorder. Advice is given as a way of conveying, for example, what is needed for a successful treatment. All these examples mostly use the objective mind to obtain a perspective on the patient's disorder.

Talk

The question may be, "How does this type of interaction affect the patient?" Talking in this manner denotes a level of professionalism and expertise, most commonly associated with a medical model form of talk therapy. However, it may fail to reach a patient at a critical time when they may be most vulnerable. Some patients may be used to this form of professional treatment and now know what to expect. "The professionals are gathering information to heal me." Or, they may find this approach discomforting where they needed to connect with another human being at this moment in some way. Regardless of its impact, it can set the tone for how treatment will proceed. It can act as an unspoken ground rule for how the mental health experience will take place. Depending on the goals of the professional, they will ask the patient to conform to the diagnosis and treatment plan.

FORMING EMPATHIC INTERACTIONS

Client Talks

There may be little information gathering at first when the client begins to talk with the counselor. Basically, what is expected from a more phenomenologically oriented counselor is to share the meaning behind a client's pain that brought him or her to the point of seeking counseling. If objective information is required by the institution, then it may be the responsibility of the counselor to make a point that counseling has not yet started until intake work is completed. Personally, I believe a counselor needs to get closure on this process with a client before sharing the pain of the client's experiences. Perhaps to wait until a therapeutic alliance is formed, especially when considering a diagnosis and treatment plan.

Your Emotion and Thought Reaction

However, when counseling has begun and the client shares their experiences, it seems important to practice some form of empathy when hearing these experiences. It means neurologically one uses those areas of the brain that will help the counselor get in touch with her or his thoughts and feelings and the impact they are having on the counselor. At this point, one might ask,

"Why are you focusing on your own feelings instead of the clients?" From a phenomenological perspective, it is important to absorb the thoughts and feelings of the client, which allows the counselor's neurological brain activities to take place. You do not only want to know about the client. You also want their thoughts to be your thoughts and their pain to be your pain.

Bracket Your Thoughts and Emotions

This next phase may show the counter-intuitive and sometimes paradoxical nature of empathy. After connecting emotionally with the client, it becomes important for you to bracket your thoughts and emotions—to put them aside, even though you may want to react back to the client. The interesting thing about empathy is that it is based on not being a reaction but an action to connect with the client, not a reaction to your emotional experiences. (Note: If you are reacting to the client personally, then we call that "identifying" with a client, not empathizing. The focus in identifying is now on you and not them.) By bracketing your thoughts and feelings, you are positioned to practice what phenomenological thinkers call a "disciplined naïveté" (Merleau-Ponty 2002; Giorgi 1983). In other words, you are making no assumptions about what the client is thinking and feeling. You are open to what emerges from this empathic interaction only in a disciplined manner where the focus is on the client.

Look through the Client's Perspective

Metaphorically speaking, it is now the process of looking through the eyes of the client. It is an attempt to enter their world and look at it through the client's lens and see the world that brought them to counseling. Sometimes this is difficult to accomplish if you are struggling with your personal emotions and are having difficulty putting them to the side. (My personal experience has been that it is easier to empathize when listening to the vulnerability of a client rather than when they are angry at the world, with me included in that world.) Regardless, if you want to connect with clients, entering their world is the gateway to that experience.

Use the Embodied Mind

It is at this point, in my view, where the phenomenological counselor becomes more sophisticated than a medical model counselor. After getting in touch with your thoughts and feelings, bracketing them, and then having looked through the client's perspective, you are now in a position to use the power of the embodied mind, namely using the prefrontal cortex, amygdala, mirror neurons, supramarginal gyrus, hippocampus, and gut—all vital processes that help the counselor accurately proceed in counseling. This makes what follows richer, more meaningful, and more open to change than an accumulation of objective information to render an expert-oriented diagnosis and treatment plan.

Talk

At this point, who knows what you will be saying to the client. However, here is some of the meaning behind the message that is being sent to the client: "I hear you. I feel your pain. I am with you in starting this process. You can trust me. We will do this together. You are not alone." Herein lies the power of empathy when interacting with clients. Even though you may be gathering information, a connection is being made, and a therapeutic alliance becomes the goal of counseling. It may be important to trust whatever you say since it is based partially on intuition, insight, or attunement.

Notice How Your Talk Affects Your Client

Do not think the process is closed regarding empathy. As you talk, start depending on your mirror neurons to make sure what you are saying is mirrored in how the client is responding. One of my problems with a medical model orientation is that the objective, expert, professional response can be assumed to be the right response, no matter what is said. However, if the client watches the expert, she or he may believe, "That is a professional response." Such a response can keep distance between the client and counselor where the counselor is the expert and the client becomes the passive "patient." In an empathic response, the focus is not on the professional but on the client and how he or she is responding to the counselor's response. At times, a professional response by an expert leaves the patient passive and disconnected even though one would judge the professional response as appropriate.

Adjust Delivery to Connect

I have observed highly competent phenomenological counselors change how and what they were saying to a client in mid-sentence because they realized what they were saying was not working. In a more phenomenological format of counseling, it may be important to gather objective information on the client but not at the expense of empathic interaction between them. The power of empathy is in its ability to connect with clients. Since a phenomenological counselor may be under pressure, in present mental health culture, to come up with a diagnosis or treatment plan before getting started, somehow an empathic connection needs to be squeezed in at some point during information gathering.

This does not mean that objective information is ignored. Accountability to insurance companies and management care institutions through progress notes, assessments, psychiatric labels, and treatment plans are presently a part of mental health culture. What it does mean is that beyond the culture there must be room for empathic client/counselor interaction. Neurologically, it makes sense to use as much of a counselor's mind when helping a client. Phenomenologically, it makes sense to use as much of the client's experiences to help the client. Empathy allows both to happen, and that is why it becomes an indispensable skill for phenomenologically oriented counselors.[3]

DISCUSSION

Some questions may arise regarding treatment from a more phenomenological perspective regarding more serious mental health problems, such as schizophrenia, schizoaffective disorder, personality disorders, developmental disabilities, substance abuse disorders, and others. Can one make a case for practicing empathy and letting problems emerge through empathic interaction with seriously mentally ill patients? Would it not be a more accurate direction to use a pharmaceutical medical model when dealing with these conditions?

If the mind of a seriously mentally ill client was presented from the brain/mind model of where problems in the brain affect disorders in the mind, the answer would be yes. However, what if the mind was considered a combination of energy and information gathering coming from the embodied brain (brain, nervous system, and the gut) combined with the interpersonal interaction with another? Then the answer may change from yes to maybe not.

Donald M. Linhorst wrote a fascinating book called *Empowering People with Severe Mental Illness: A Practical Guide* (2006) where he spend s time describing the benefits of empowering seriously mentally ill patients. In numerous areas, it may be beneficial to include these patients in the decision-making process and negotiations concerning their mental illness. Any process that prepares patients to participate more effectively in activities that increase their power, control, or influence can be considered empowering (Zimmerman 2000). Empowerment for seriously mentally ill patients may include: increased confidence, improved social skills, greater knowledge of resources, and stabilization of psychiatric symptoms (Linhorst 2006).

In present mental health culture, serious mental health problems are mostly looked at as medical problems. This is based on psychiatrists treating the patient as though they have a medical illness based on symptoms of a specific mental disorder, such as schizophrenia. A more phenomenological approach looks at serious mental health problems as something the client is experiencing or going through and what can be changed within that experience that would empower the client to live a more fruitful life. The present culture of mental health may not be willing to give up a strictly medical model view of these serious mental problems, especially where drugs are concerned. However, from the experience of the client, their empowerment may be a crucial element in their ongoing struggle with, for example, schizophrenia.

Empathy lies at the heart of a phenomenological model where listening carefully to the needs of a client who is in serious mental pain can emerge a therapeutic alliance where empowerment in decision-making, increased confidence, improved social skills, greater knowledge of resources, and stabilization of psychiatric symptoms will improve their mental health experience. For psychiatrists, it is the disorder of the patients where their focus lies. For the patient, it is the experience of going through the disorder where their focus lies. Empathy opens the door for empowerment of seriously mentally ill patients, and where a patient's rights are protected, allowing them to be the unrecognized experts in what they are going through (Ladd and Churchill 2012).

Does this mean that a more phenomenologically oriented model should replace a medical model when dealing with serious mental illness problems? It is doubtful that this replacement will happen or should happen anytime soon. What it may mean is that a phenomenological form of counseling may be a crucial addition in capturing the client's experience of going through, for example, schizophrenia—by acting as a whole person and participating as an unrecognized expert. Again, empathy acts as a gateway to the severely mentally troubled clients to be empowered and to face the experience of living in this world.

NOTES

1. In the twenty-five years that I ran the Holistic Health and Wellness Clinic, a mental health facility, the clinic had guidelines to keep the business of mental health separate from the practice of counseling and therapy. At times, another professional would gather information from clients instead of the counselors assigned for counseling. Or, the counselors would gather information but make it very clear that counseling had not yet begun. This helped client and counselor establish a therapeutic alliance when the practice of counseling began. Peter D. Ladd, Mental Health Clinical Practice, 1987 through 2015.

2. This is one reason that I believe motivational interviewing is effective. Neurologically, it gathers information and at the same time makes an empathic connection with the client. Such action helps steer the counselor more towards what is important for the client than trying to meet the needs of the counselor. The activity is more in line with a phenomenological approach to counseling. Miller, William, and Steven Rollnick. 2012. *Motivational Interviewing: Helping People Change.* New York, NY: Guilford Press, 1–10.

3. This is as I stated in Chapter 1 regarding the phenomenologically oriented mental health clinic that I ran for many years. Objective information was initially taken for purposes of insurance and record-keeping, but no diagnosis or treatment plan was developed until after a therapeutic alliance was formed with the client. Even then, the client had input into both the

diagnosis and treatment plan. Peter D. Ladd, Mental Health Clinical Practice, 1987 through 2015.

Chapter Six

Insightful Revelations

Insight links the past, present, and future. Insight means integrating cortical representation of autobiographical memory stores and limbic firing that gives emotional texture to the emerging themes of our present awareness, life story, and image of the future (Siegel 2010). In other words, insight puts together a collection of memories along with spurts of emotion to create an emotional meaning to what the client is experiencing regarding the present, past life stories, and images of the future.

From a phenomenological perspective, insight helps clients understand how events in their past are currently influencing their current thoughts, emotions, and behaviors along with an understanding of how these insights can affect future events. Insights not only help with awareness but also with meaning during a counseling session. Insight connects the past, present, and future so that a client considers more than an experience about the present and to think about during talk therapy. Past experiences and possible future experiences add meaning to what is happening in the client's life during counseling. Insight makes present problems more complex when considering how a client's experiences have influenced those present problems and how those same problems will influence the client's future.

NEUROSCIENCE AND INSIGHT

Before getting started in understanding neuroscience and insight, it may be important to think about what might be bringing clients to counseling in the first place. Much of what is practiced from day-to-day are habits coordinated in the striatum, which is located deep beneath the cortex where it forms part of the basal ganglia (McKay 2017). The striatum is richly connected to the prefrontal cortex (involved in higher-order thinking, feeling, and sensing) and to the midbrain. The midbrain provides input from dopamine-containing neurons (brain cells) (Roeper 2013). Dopamine is a brain chemical that is strongly associated with creating positive feelings related to reward and events of emotional significance (Bergland 2012). From a medical model perspective, a malfunctioning striatum may have implications when habits become disordered, such as obsessive-compulsive behaviors and addiction (McKay 2017). Therefore, habits may be considered beneficial most of the time, such as learning to walk, driving a car, and so forth. So, for clients, it may be unsuccessful habits that bring clients to counseling. I call some of these habits "disorders."[1]

These unsuccessful and painful habits are discussed during talk therapy. Sometimes they are resolved through more step-by-step procedures. Other times, insight occurs when a client suddenly reinterprets something discussed in counseling that produces nonobvious, original interpretation of a problem. This can take the form of a solution to a problem (an "*aha!*" moment) and a comprehension of an experience or recognition of an ambiguous perception of a client problem that can point to its solution (Kounios and Jung-Beeman 2009).

To see how insight affects counseling, let us compare two types of problem-solving that are found in a pharmaceutical medical model and a more phenomenological model. For the most part, a pharmaceutical medical model solves problems by incrementally processing information. For example, the information gathered from a patient during intake will be added to the information gathered from the psychiatrist, which will be added to the information gathered by the therapist. This is how a patient's file is accumulated for solving mental problems. It is a form of problem-solving where the focus is on visually looking over the material connected to the patient's problems and drawing conclusions as to what must be done for the patient. It is this incremental collection of data and processing it where conclusions are made as to what should be the treatment plan and direction for talk therapy.

Solving problems in talk therapy through insight is different. Insight is the sudden awareness of the solution to a problem with little or no conscious access to the processing of information leading up to that solution. This type of problem-solving becomes most effective when the therapist sets the stage for insights to happen spontaneously. Important insights may happen more often in therapy when the therapist tries to form a therapeutic alliance by practicing empathy and where the therapist uses her or his intuition while being closely attuned to the client. Under these conditions, client solutions to problems may "pop out" unexpectedly during therapy.

Neurologically, this happens when signals in the right anterior superior temporal gyrus transmit through the right anterior superior temporal lobe a gamma response beginning at approximately the moment when the solution reveals itself in therapy (Bowden, Jung-Beeman, Fleck, and Kounios 2005).

Therefore, insight reflects the cognitive phenomenon of solutions becoming available in a sudden, discrete fashion. Some experts believe it can be identified as an important characteristic of creative thought (Bowden, Jung-Beeman, Fleck, and Kounios 2005).

If I may speak metaphorically, insight is like a virus. It lies dormant until at some spontaneous moment it reveals itself with clarity and purpose. In some respects, insight is more likely to emerge in both the client and therapist when the bond between them is strong and the collaboration is meaningful. However, in my experience, clients having moments of insight do not only happen in the therapist's office. A client could be walking down the street and suddenly he or she knows what to do to solve their mental problems. Here is an example of insight:

Fred had been in counseling for months after the divorce proceedings took place between himself and his wife. During this time, he struggled with loss, anger, and sadness; however, nothing seemed to help him. He wanted to move on from this sad experience in his life but could not seem to let go of it. His counselor did her best to listen to his sadness, anger, and loss and stayed closely attuned to his feelings as the number of sessions increased with no results.

One day Fred was walking down the street and a picture of what he needed to do popped into his mind. Fred went to this old wooden bridge near where he lived, and inside his coat was a small bottle of champagne. He took a moment at the bridge to drink the champagne and then threw the empty bottle in the river. Next, he took off his wedding ring and threw it in the river as well.

When he returned to his therapist, Fred seemed different. He was more relaxed and more confident in himself. He told his therapist about what he had done and thanked her for helping him come to this highly meaningful decision in his life. He said that without her help, he could have spent years stuck in the black hole that he had dug for himself. The therapist thanked Fred for his honesty and the effort that finally led to his growth and change. After Fred left, the therapist sat for many minutes trying to recount what had happened during therapy. She concluded that the empathy, attunement, and intuitive decisions that went into the therapeutic alliance for both finally spilled over into an answer for Fred.

From this story, one could make the argument that Fred and his therapist spent more time emotionally connecting over the problem than trying to solve it. Neurologically, these types of connections lower feelings of being threatened in the hypothalamus, which governs the body's hormonal stress response and increases the possibility for effective problem-solving. The hypothalamus is the "H" of the hypothalamic-pituitary-adrenal (HPA) axis, which mediates the release of the stress hormone cortisol that may interfere with the ability to focus on therapy problems (Cavanagh 2013). Instead, Fred and his therapist formed a therapeutic alliance that created a bond between them and added to Fred's ability to have insight into his wife leaving him.

This allowed Fred to trust the therapy process and come to a point where all that was shared between client and therapist would eventually surface in the form of an answer to his problem. The fact that the "*aha!* moment" came when he was not in a therapy session lends itself to realizing that Fred's embodied brain was working with little focus on incremental, step-by-step cognitive problem-solving going on within his mind. Like a virus, his thoughts about what to do regarding letting go of his anger, sadness, and loss remained dormant until it reached a critical mass where spontaneously he had an insight as to what needed to be done.

One of the differences between a pharmaceutical medical model and a phenomenological model is in how problems are solved in therapy. A medical model focuses on a step-by-step gathering of information until a calculated decision can be made partially based on probability regarding what to do for the patient with mental illness. A phenomenological model stays attuned, empathizes, and allows intuition to help in resolving a mental health problem. It also gathers information more intuitively until some form of insight emerges that helps in resolving the client's problems. This means that phenomenological therapy relies more on trust than on control. This is in contrast to a more medical model therapist who tries to control problem-solving at each step along the way to patient recovery.

The question may be asked, "Do symptoms have to be controlled while a patient is in crisis?" A pharmaceutically based medical model certainly has had success when patients are in crisis. Psychotropic drugs are given. Counseling techniques are used to reduce symptoms, where both are under the control of a mental health professional. However, when it comes to dealing with what is meaningful to clients, control does not necessarily empower clients to find meaning in their lives. Therefore, the medical model seems to deal effectively with crisis and maintaining stability.

However, not all of talk therapy is crisis counseling, and not all clients are looking for stability. Once a client is stabilized, there is a world of possibilities for growth and change. It is my opinion that such a world is more effectively approached from a whole person perspective. The neurological process where a client feels comfortable, safe, and with close therapeutic support seems to be where problem-solving based on that "spontaneous moment" can take place. Where a combination of past, present, and future experiences come together, and it is where something insightful pops into the mind of the client or the therapist and gives direction and guidance to what comes next. Our minds are a complex organism that not only has a step-by-step method for solving problems, but it also has a method where information comes together all at once in an insightful resolution to client problems.

PHENOMENOLOGY AND INSIGHT

The famous philosopher Maurice Merleau-Ponty wrote an article entitled *Cezanne's Doubt* where he described how the artist Paul Cézanne, when painting, would look at the canvas over one hundred times before he could finish it (Merleau-Ponty 1992). Here is an artist who practiced insightful problem-solving. On the other hand, on vacation, I once bought a kit that helped me paint by the numbers. It was a step-by-step process where the directions guided me from one stroke on the canvas to the next stroke. Unfortunately, the vacation turned out to be more memorable than my artistic creation.

When you look at comparing medical model talk therapy with a more phenomenological model regarding how each solves problems, a considerable difference stands out. A medical model focuses on patient symptoms by controlling the process in a more step-by-step fashion where experts can control and direct what problems need solving and empirically focus on what needs attention by referencing the *DSM-5*. A phenomenological model focuses on the whole person by allowing the connection between client and counselor to look at the client's problems from many different angles and experiences. This process is used until a problem is resolved through the emergence of an insightful moment where it is clear to the client and counselor what needs to be done next. In some respects, phenomenological-oriented talk therapists are more similar to artists than scientists, and the procedures they use are based more on a human science rather than natural science (Giorgi 1970).

Some of the criticism that comes from a phenomenological model of talk therapy is that a more holistic form of talk therapy can show no empirical evidence that it is effective. The question one may ask is, "Do we want to reduce human experience to a point where it is measurable at the expense of understanding a phenomenon when it reveals itself in real time?" In many respects, human experience can be distorted by using natural scientific methods and statistical probabilities. In my opinion, through natural scientific methodology, many of the nuances that make us human are left unappreciated on the cutting-room floor.

However, the idea of a therapeutic alliance has been researched and shown as one of the most effective processes in talk therapy (Hansen 2016; Cronin, Brand, and Mattanah 2014). Furthermore, insightful problem-solving in talk therapy does not base solving problems on a hunch or a guess. Neurologically, it is a different form of solving problems than incrementally processing information. There are many perceptual attempts to understand the past, present, and future regarding the client's mental health problems while the therapist stays attuned to the client and forms a meaningful collaboration that hopefully leads to some insight—some spontaneous moment where the problem being discussed is different in some way.

If talk therapists are looking for the legitimacy of this process, do not only turn to psychological greats such as Viktor Frankl or Carl Rogers (Frankl 1967; Rogers 2003). Turn to Albert Einstein, who based many of his greatest discoveries not on his incremental problem-solving abilities but on countlessly thinking about his theories, sometimes for years, until some insightful revelation appeared (Norton 2016). This leads to the reality that, in some respects, insightful problem-solving requires emotional commitment, for it can be emotionally draining and a lot of work. First, it requires both client and therapist to discuss the present problem from many different angles and in numerous ways. That is until, neurologically, signals in the right anterior superior temporal gyrus transmit through the right anterior superior temporal lobe where a gamma response begins at approximately the moment when the solution reveals itself in therapy—and that process can be exhausting. However, this neurological process is a matter of cognition, not a guess. The client and therapist are dwelling on a problem with the commitment to collaborate on it until the past, present, and future combine in making the emergent insight recognizable and accurate. Take the following story as an example of insight.

Jennifer had been to numerous psychiatrists and psychologists regarding her anxiety. She had taken drugs for it, tried techniques to reduce it, and any number of other attempts to deal with it. None of these attempts worked, even the psychotropic drugs. In a state of desperation, she called a more holistic mental health counselor who welcomed her and treated her situation with the utmost respect. Jennifer and her therapist would spend many sessions talking about her anxiety and why she felt so confused about it. There seemed to be no place in her life where she could say implicitly that the problem was this issue or that one. The more she talked about her anxiety, the more it seemed not to make sense to both her and her therapist.

After numerous sessions, her therapist suddenly felt the urge to ask this question, "Has anyone that you have seen for anxiety ever described how anxiety works?" The answer was no. Her therapist then began to show that it starts with uncertainty followed by a person narrowing his or her focus on it by incrementally looking for step-by-step answers to the problem. Her counselor stated that one of the problems with anxiety is that it was counterintuitive (the more you try to solve it the worse it gets). The result of this type of unsuccessful problem-solving was to constantly worry, which leads to symptoms developing and finally finding yourself in an uncontrolled state of crisis.

Over the next week, Jennifer thought about what the therapist had said. When she arrived for her next appointment, she told the therapist that three days ago after eating dinner, all her anxiety began to leave her. What emerged as she thought about it was this insight that she had anxiety about having anxiety, and when the therapist described how anxiety worked, Jennifer's uncertainty had lifted, and her worrying was gone. She commented that previous professionals kept trying to solve her anxiety based on the symptoms she was presenting and trying to solve her problem through a step-by-step treatment plan that seemed to cause more anxiety instead of connecting with and talking to her. The phenomenological-oriented therapist developed a meaningful dialogue and let insight emerge as the therapy progressed. Ironically, the therapist was not around when the insight happened. Jennifer took full ownership of it but recognized the therapist as an important collaborator in developing this insight.

In this story, it was not by chance that Jennifer liberated herself from anxiety. She adopted a way of problem-solving used by many successful musicians, artists, scientists, leaders, and therapists—a way of solving problems that is neurologically sound. In the current mental health culture, this form of problem-solving seems lost—too mystical, poetic, or artistic. This form of thinking and practicing therapy seems on the fringes of a dominant medical model that places practices such as talking about things but not really doing anything to help mental health patients. The present pharmaceutically based medical model at times flattens human complexity for the sake of diagnosis and shows indifference to the humanistic, holistic, and nuanced perspective of the client (Egan 2012). It may be that experts in the field of talk therapy rely on empirical, precise, statistical, and symptomatic problem-solving with clients, and this is sometimes at the expense of experiential, comprehensive, meaningful, holistic, and insightful problem-solving made in collaboration between client and therapist (Ladd and Churchill 2012).

INCREMENTAL PROBLEM-SOLVING

Identify the Problem

Much of what is involved in a more incremental problem-solving methodology can be found in most natural scientific research. Usually there is an attempt to find the background that makes up the problem. For example, in a more medical model form of talk therapy, this begins with an understanding of the client's history. Are there any previous reports of mental problems? Has any assessment been done that clarifies the history of mental problems? Are there any previous diagnoses that shed light on current problems? The purpose of this type of inquiry is to form a foundation for making a hypothesis regarding what action can be taken. In medical model counseling, this information and purpose are gathered to eventually develop a treatment plan. It also gives the mental health institution a record of what has already happened to the patient and what is the current amount of information with how to proceed with a diagnosis and treatment plan.

Define Goals

In most incremental problem-solving, the goals to proceed are clearly defined or the eventual problem-solving plan could drift into unnecessary goals that do not match the evidence put forward by the gathering of information and the assessment of this information. In a medical model, defining goals is based on mental health history, current presenting of mental symptoms, and a diagnosis that matches those symptoms. From a more phenomenological model, defining goals this early in the process may be beneficial if the patient is in crisis and safety becomes the main concern, but it may be premature for fully understanding the problem from a whole person perspective. Again, as I have said before, some people will not reveal their most compelling mental problems until a therapeutic alliance is formed with a mental health professional. However, to remain in control of the entire medical model process, historical groundwork and a diagnosis of symptoms must be made to come up with a treatment plan that becomes the guideline for doing therapy.

Brainstorming

The checking on the success or failure of any problem-solving venture may require some form of checking in on the progress taking place in solving the problem. In medical model mental health procedures, checking in sometimes requires a case management meeting to discuss the client where different points of view can add to the ongoing assessment of the patient's progress. As someone who has spent years running mental health clinics, it seems reasonable to involve others in this form of brainstorming. Others can look at the patient's file and add information from their respective points of view. However, from a more phenomenological point of view, unfortunately, there seems to be one point of view that is missing—it is the point of view of the patient. Even when the therapist reports back the views of the patient through progress notes and other written devices, they still may not be a part of the conversation that determines their mental health future. Informing clients of the views of others has consistently worked, in my experience, whether it is being involved in discussing the plan of treatment or in forming a diagnosis.

Assess Alternatives

In a more incremental method of problem-solving after discussing the plan with others, professionals are now in a position to change a plan that is not working. Here is where ideas can be incorporated into what also needs to be considered regarding solving the problem. This seems to apply to most medical model problem-solving where assessments are made that may change the manner of treatment taking place with any given patient. However, from a medical model using only an incremental problem-solving style, it assumes that gathering accurate information can only come from this type of problem-solving. From a more phenomenological viewpoint, this is viewed as an inaccurate assumption. The mind of a patient can also supply valuable information through insight gathered while intimately connected to the therapist. This information may not be available through incremental problem-solving, but it may be vital for the growth and change of the patient.

Act Out a Solution

The last step in using incremental problem-solving is to act out the solution to the problem. If the gathering of information was accurate, and the goals were on target, along with brainstorming alternatives and finally assessing the problem accurately, then acting out the solution should resolve the problem. In a medical model method of incremental problem-solving, this method seems the most orderly way and a method that can be controlled by mental health experts. However, it may not be the most efficient method for helping patients with their mental health problems. The mental health solution from a medical model focuses on symptoms reduction and symptoms maintenance. The rate of patients staying on drugs and returning for therapy, in a medical model, may be orderly, but one could question whether it is efficient regarding patients returning to therapy.

However, such a problem-solving solution can be profitable, especially for big pharma. By focusing on symptoms reduction and symptoms maintenance, pharmaceutical companies have created an industry that may not be looking for other problem-solving methods, especially those based on growth and change. A phenomenological model based on growth and change is based on solving problems through more insightful and creative methods that are conceived by the client and not the experts, and this may be one of the reasons insightful problem-solving is not more popular with strictly medical model professionals.

INSIGHTFUL REVELATIONS

Focus on Uncovering the Problem

It seems more difficult to focus on uncovering problems in talk therapy without having formed a therapeutic alliance. That does not mean that during the building of a relationship between therapist and client that information gathering is any different than that found in incremental problem-solving. A baseline of information seems important, if for nothing else than to get a frame of reference as to who is talking to the therapist. It may be how the information is gathered where the difference becomes apparent. In incremental problem-solving, information is gathered in therapy by the therapist asking preconceived questions that follow a specific format created before meeting with the client or directed by the therapist during initial meetings. From a more insightful form of problem-solving, the therapist may simply ask, "So tell me about yourself." This allows the client to decide what information they would like to initially discuss and which information they initially would decide to withhold. Though this presents a less controllable set of circumstances for the therapist, it empowers the client to set the tone and the pace for how the sessions will proceed. (Unfortunately, the business of mental health needs more standardized information to be perceived as credible. During therapy, I am not sure this is the case.)

It also sets unspoken rules that are beneficial when asking someone to reveal their deepest and most vulnerable experiences. Here are some of the unspoken rules that may develop when empowering clients while focusing on uncovering the problem:

- Clients set the limits to what they are willing to share at any given moment and at any given time.
- As your counselor, I am not here to gather information for judgment but to listen to your story.
- Your experiences are important and have meaning.
- I am not looking for symptoms but want to know you as a person.

There are probably others, but these alone set the stage for where the therapy is heading and what roles client and therapist play in these sessions. There is one more unspoken rule that must be added after a therapeutic alliance is formed: "From here on out, we will be collaborating as equals by combining your experiences with my expertise."

Perceive Multiple Avenues

Forming a therapeutic alliance now puts the client and therapist in a position to look at the client's experiences from many different avenues. This is quite different than a more incremental problem-solving medical model where the client's experiences are looked at from the angle of a therapist searching for evidence that backs up his or her treatment plan. This form of selective perceiving of the problem becomes only effective if the original hypothesis (diagnose and treatment plan) are accurate. It is the agreed upon angle of the psychiatrist, talk therapist, and whoever else agrees to the treatment plan.

From a more phenomenological talk therapy perspective, allowing many avenues of perception to be explored creates a climate of diversity. It develops possibilities in the mind of the client that any one of these avenues is possible. For the therapist, such multiple avenue perceptions also create possibilities for the therapist in how to respond to the client with attunement and intuitive decision-making. Such offering of many avenues of possibilities to both client and therapist allow experiences from the past, present, and future to intermix if or when they become appropriate to talk about. Such dialogue in phenomenological talk therapy allows the experience of the client as a whole person to emerge and it allows the therapist to perceive the client as a whole person.

Dwell on These Avenues

Here is where the true nature of insightful revelations has the opportunity to take place. There is now the potential for an established commitment by the client and the therapist to happen both inside and outside of therapy. Neurologically, the mind is in a position to take these avenues and simplify them, to make sense of them, and to dwell on them. This happens not in any systematic way but by letting the right anterior superior temporal gyrus do its job. From a neurological viewpoint, the brain is trying to simplify all these avenues uncovered in talk therapy to something that is more manageable. That is why meditation, mindfulness, doing one thing at a time (dwelling on client problems), and avoiding distractions (being taught counseling techniques when necessary) all help in this dwelling process.

Trust the Process

Many talk therapists have heard the statement, "trust the process," but do many of them exactly know what that means? From a medical model of talk therapy point of view, such a statement may be too disorganized to control. The therapist needs control in performing the duties of a treatment plan, and much of a medical model is based on control. However, from a more phenomenologically based therapy model, the main overriding principle is based on trust. This form of therapy is asking the client and the therapist to know each other and form a bond and trust where that bond will take them.

It asks when dwelling on all the avenues that have been considered during therapy, that the more we trust each other and the more we focus on the client's recovery that eventually there will be some important insight into the client's problems. The cognitive and emotional bond through mirror neurons in both participant's brains and the emotional responses from the bodies of both, through sharing attuned emotional and physical bonds, will add to the insightful revelations that may take place. In some respects, "trust the process" is synonymous with "trust the workings of the brain."

Insightful Moments Emerge

At this point is where these processes come together through client and therapist focusing on uncovering the problem, by perceiving multiple avenues, dwelling on these avenues, and, finally, trusting the process to form insightful problem-solving where "spontaneous moments" can emerge. Such moments are not created by chance or by luck or by a guess. They are formed around an alternative method of problem-solving used by artists, musicians, creative scientists, and by phenomenological and humanistic talk therapists. Having insight in the therapy process can be a profound revelation. It requires work combined with trust. Working closely with each other in therapy and trusting each other to find a way out of pain may be one of the most powerful experiences that talk therapy has to offer clients. It is the ultimate form of integration. Ironically, though it is not organized by natural scientific standards, it is remarkably efficient. Growing and changing as a whole person rather than constantly being treated for symptoms reduction seems a more efficient method for solving client problems.

DISCUSSION

It seems that both incremental problem-solving and insightful revelations have a place in talk therapy. It does not make sense not to use both when helping patients/clients. There is much that can be gained from using a medical model, especially when a patient is in crisis. It does not make sense that a patient, when in crisis, should wait for an insightful answer to emerge. The main goal at this point, like in any crisis, is the theme of safety where the patient is safe from self-harm, safe from getting worse, and safe from facing a world that they may not be able to face without some help, whether that help is through psychotropic drugs or a controlled regiment of counseling techniques.

Having said that, it also does not make sense to keep treating the patient as though they were in crisis when they may be ready to find themselves through some form of growth and change. However, it also does not make sense from the very beginning of talk therapy to put clients through the same medical model procedures at a point where they can gain from knowing themselves. Or, where they have the opportunities and possibilities to change portions of their identity and meaning in their lives. Unfortunately, such a process is more difficult to find in a strictly medical model of therapy.

One might suggest that an assessment be done with patients/clients to determine for people seeking mental health services as to what type of approach is appropriate, crisis intervention or growth and change.[2] As professionals, we cannot assume that when people come for mental health services that all of them are in crisis or that all are looking for symptoms reduction.

Conversely, we also cannot assume that someone in deep crisis should immediately seek out growth and change. Finally, it may be in chronic situations regarding a disorder that drug therapy needs to be extended while clients seek out growth and change. However, there is no reason not to do both.

NOTES

1. Personally, I have thought for a long time that the experience of mental disorders seemed more associated with unsuccessful habits rather than fitting the description of mental disorders. First, mental disorders are not only mental. They are more than that. Secondly, they are not a disorder but rather they create disorder in the client's experience. On the other hand, habits fit more closely with neuropathways in the brain that neurologically correspond to what is happening in the outside world. Peter D. Ladd. 2013. *Knowledge versus Wisdom in a* DSM *Diagnosis. A Person-Centered Perspective.* Washington, DC: American Counseling Association.

2. I would suggest some form of motivational interviewing be developed that could direct a client/patient toward an effective therapeutic model that meets their needs. The medical model idea that one-size-fits-all seems a bit outdated when trying to create a climate of diversity in how to approach mental health procedures. However, it may turn out that the solution to this issue needs be decided whether this is a therapy problem or a political problem. Therapeutically, for me, it makes sense to have options for those who seek mental health help. However, politically it may be too big of a business move for big pharma and the psychiatric associations to accept. Peter Ladd 2017.

Chapter Seven

Selfless Acts

NEUROSCIENCE AND SELFLESS ACTS

Phenomenological talk therapy is filled with selfless acts. The relationship itself in counseling focuses on the interaction between client and counselor. It is a nurturing relationship where the client is the person being nurtured and the counselor is the nurturer. Counselors as nurturers, by definition, create a comfortable and safe environment so that clients can feel free to explore the areas where suffering is taking place. From a neurological perspective, this type of relationship is more common in our existence than experts believed only a few years ago.

It is now being proposed by some researchers that the traditional mode of people being selfish and then forcing themselves to be generous might be wrong. New research demonstrates that people enjoy being generous, but in certain circumstances, they overcome a displeasure to be selfish (Zaki, López, and Mitchell 2014). For example, the anxious mother would love to spend more time with her children, but anxiety keeps her self-centered and self-serving. We may be more inclined to be generous with others unless certain circumstances change our behavior in favor of selfishness.

In counseling, selfless acts of the counselor through such experiences as showing positive regard to clients is aimed at creating a climate of generosity. Client and counselor begin to share experiences that help them during therapy. Neurologically, present studies demonstrate that social cognition and connections through the dorsomedial prefrontal cortex (dmPFC) can predict unselfish behavior. Research has found that the response from the dorsomedial prefrontal cortex predicted subsequent altruistic behavior based on when a situation is equitable between two people. Under these circumstances, when the situation is fair and equitable, people tend to be unselfish (Waytz, Zaki, and Mitchell 2012).

What does this mean for more humanistic, phenomenological talk therapy? Its connotation is that positive regard, compassion, empathy, appreciation, and other emotional connections between client and counselor may be regarded as natural phenomena. Clients perceiving a counseling session as fair and equitable may be more accessible to healing. These emotional experiences between client and counselor are not a technique or a plan. When shared by the counselor, it becomes a natural process where a client may experience some form of growth and change.

Having emphasized the positive through selfless acts, it may be hard to believe in a somewhat cynical world where, neurologically, we are more inclined to be selfless and caring than negative and cautious (Breuning 2016). All things being equal, practicing selfless actions should be more predominant than selfish and fearful behavior. Unfortunately, in today's world, all things are not equal. Neurologically, we are more prepared for negative, tragic events than positive ones. In such a world, there are times when we can be shocked by current events or experience negative emotions around us that subjugate selfless acts. In these times, areas of the middle brain will shoot cortisol and adrenaline through our bodies, making us respond as though we were naturally inclined to be cautious, negative, and selfish. Survival as humans on this planet has taught us that being vigilant and careful when letting our guard down is not a bad idea. However, it may be important to realize that being negative is not necessarily all that makes up our given nature (Hanson 2013).[1] This may be why it is important to develop a dialogue that accents the positive with clients who may not only be in mental pain but also live in a world where pain is no stranger.

Here is a story where very little was done regarding a treatment plan or the use of counseling techniques. Mark had a saying that he shared with his clients: "I will hang in there with you if you hang in there with me." Little did he know that his saying would be tested over the next few months. John was an Afghanistan War veteran who had experienced severe trauma and who fell into trouble with alcohol and anger issues. He went to numerous centers that treated veteran's issues from a medical model, but no one could help him with either of his problems. Fortunately, he was well-respected in the small town where he lived, which helped John stay out of jail for bar fights and drunk driving.

Mark, his counselor, was one of the few people John trusted, and Mark helped John on numerous occasions by vouching for him with police and other authorities. One day while counseling at the town's mental health clinic, Mark got a call from the police saying that John was locked in his home, drunk, and with a pistol in his hand. The police had surrounded the house and were waiting for Mark to show up.

When Mark arrived, he saw John sitting at the kitchen table, gun in hand, and talking profusely about issues considered dangerous. Mark said to John, "You probably could shoot me, but I wish you would talk to me. It is up to you." John decided on the latter, and they talked for a few hours. When they were done, the police told John he would spend a night in the hospital for safety reasons. Mark went with him until John was settled for the night. The next day, John went to Mark for counseling. He vented all the horrific events that happened in Afghanistan, and he cried continuously. For the next six months, Mark saw John for counseling, which was basically John venting and Mark listening.

Two years later, John wrote to Mark and told him that he had entered graduate school and wanted to thank him for being there and treating him as an equal. A bond had been created, and many of the selfless acts demonstrated by Mark had changed John's life—according to John. On reflection, Mark could not remember any specific technique being used or any specific goal being stated in the counseling sessions. John simply was responding to Mark's selfless attitude towards him. That was a few years ago, and now John is helping other veterans with their problems.

PHENOMENOLOGY AND SELFLESS ACTS

It may be surprising to many people, but being selfless takes less effort than being selfish (Turner 2016). It is easier to strengthen human relations than to spend exhaustive energy tearing them down. Even when it seems easier to tear down a relationship, sometimes just one selfless act can build it up again. We are social creatures, and our brains have evolved to be social and selfless, even though at times the climate or culture of our society makes us exhaust ourselves with selfish behavior. Sometimes we become defensive while acting out in a world that appears fearful and dangerous.

We have observed selfless behavior in times of crisis, such as during hurricanes, mass shootings, and other tragic events. People reach out in a selfless show of solidarity. However, it should not take a catastrophic event for people to reach out in a selfless manner. This puts into perspective the challenge to the talk therapist in counseling clients in an imperfect world. It may be that beyond all the effort put into being a mental health professional, the training may not be enough. This should not be the type of work where becoming an expert is the goal.

Here is a comparison shared at a conference on humanistic psychology: "For the surgeon, the most important instrument is the scalpel; for the dentist, it is the drill; for mental health professionals, it is ourselves." The selfless acts of Mark in helping John in the example story shows a quality that should be sought after when entering the mental health profession. In a more humanistic, experiential form of talk therapy, selfless acts seem indispensable.

Take for example the selfless act of generosity. Generous people begin with the belief that including others in goals and aspirations may be a more desirable and productive enterprise (Wilson 2013; Marts 1966). The practice of being sensitive to the needs of others can create an unspoken rule; that generosity can be a vital component within any group pursuing a common goal (Ladd and Blanchfield 2016). Another point that is vital to talk therapists is the paradox of sharing. Paradoxically, the more the therapist practices selfless acts, the more the client becomes invested in the counseling process—paradoxically, the more you give, the more you get in return.

One last point on generosity, it is not only based on giving to others; one also needs to be accessible to them. In the story regarding Mark and John, John realized that Mark would be there for him. He realized that Mark's role was more than a job. It was an avocation. Beyond all the learning to become a talk therapist, it is the issue of how therapists see themselves. How deeply involved is the therapist in themselves when doing this kind of activity?

We have already observed how mirror neurons in the brain of a therapist begin to imitate a picture of what the client is experiencing. This act of empathy by the therapist can be viewed by the client as a selfless act. There may be no self-centered judgments being made or analysis being performed. The selfless act by the therapist to empathize creates a bond where the client is more receptive to the counseling process. Selfless acts help in creating a meaningful dialogue, and empathy creates the climate for that process to happen during counseling.

In contrast, the client may have entered counseling being self-centered and self-serving. One of the side effects of such disorders as anxiety, depression, attention deficit disorder, obsessive-compulsive disorder, panic disorder, and many others is the constant focus on one's self. In all fairness, such a focus may not be intentional. However, the pain and lack of certainty that is involved in these disorders make it difficult, at times, to be selfless and other-directed. One of the intentions of a more phenomenologically based mental health counselor may be to help clients stop thinking about themselves. Thus the importance of meaningful dialogue becomes where the counseling experience is not about the client but the collaboration that takes place between client and counselor.

The phenomenon of positive regard is another selfless act that needs to be mentioned in a more phenomenological form of talk therapy. Carl Rogers spoke about unconditional positive regard in many of his books on counseling and therapy (1951). From a neurological perspective, positive regard is more than being nice to someone. It creates the phenomenon of equity and fairness in the minds of those receiving it. For example, the response from the dorsomedial prefrontal cortex of a client from unconditional positive regard given by the counselor may create a more selfless attitude in the client when discussing counseling problems. How is this possible? Neurologically, it may put less effort on your brain to focus outside yourself while suffering through anxiety, depression, and other disorders when all things are equal (Allen and Suttie 2015).

PHENOMENOLOGY AND COMPASSION FATIGUE

Before getting into a phenomenological description of selfless acts, let us go to the dark side for a practicing mental health professional. One of the dangers for those experiential therapists who pride themselves in practicing selfless actions with their clients is the phenomenon of "compassion fatigue." Ironically, compassion fatigue can come from practicing too many selfless acts when counseling clients. The following is a story to make this point.

Janet was one of the most popular counselors at the mental health clinic. She seemed to have the best results with clients, which was attributed to her selfless attitude. The administration realized her value to the agency and asked that many of the more difficult cases be assigned to her. Janet was not a complainer, even when her caseload became well beyond what was reasonable. Her exposure to secondhand stress made her work much harder than usual, but her commitment to clients and her selfless attitude kept her going. From the day she entered graduate school, she had a strong commitment to helping others and her beliefs about helping had not wavered over the years.

However, at one point in her busy schedule, she started to feel tired and rundown. Her selfless beliefs kept her going, but her body began sending a different message. She found herself in counseling having difficulty focusing on her clients while spending more time focusing on how exhausted she was feeling during these sessions. Over time, the profession she loved and was committed to had become incrementally more difficult. It took time for her to admit that she was becoming emotionally exhausted with the work. However, her selfless beliefs were strong, which encouraged her to hang in there and keep helping clients.

At night, it was a different story. There seemed to be a war going on between her selfless beliefs and her emotionally exhausted body. This confusion was highly stressful, producing confusion over her beliefs and her emotions. She still believed in her clients, but when approaching them, she felt resistant to their stories. With time, her physical health began winning over her strong beliefs as a mental health counselor. When clients would arrive for counseling, she felt a sense of frustration when they shared their problems. Some of her responses became unrecognizable to her, such as, "Why don't you just get over it?" or "You need to get moving on solving your problems."

At some point, Janet began to resent the process of counseling. She was burnt out but refused to admit it.

Over time, people noticed that Janet was thinking more about herself than the progress being made with clients. She made constant complaints about how lazy some clients acted when asked to practice a technique or complete an assignment. Eventually, she began to feel physically ill. She went to the administration and stated that she wanted to resign. When asked about why she came to such a conclusion, her answer was, "When clients come to me, I feel sick to my stomach listening to their problems." They recommended that she seek counseling. Janet eventually took a few weeks off, and then she took their advice. Within six months, her beliefs were restored, and her physical health returned. In the final analysis, she realized that sometimes you could be too good for your own good. That being too responsible is irresponsible.

In this story, Janet went from a superstar to a failure in counseling. Her selflessness had turned into resentment. To quote an unknown source, "You cannot give water from an empty bucket." And Janet's bucket was empty. The following is the phenomenological pattern that eventually led to Janet's seeking counseling. It is called compassion fatigue.

Compassion Fatigue

Exposure to Secondhand Stress

Usually, compassion fatigue starts with overexposure to secondhand stress. This means you do not have to experience stress directly but simply show compassion for others going through stress. Each time you do this, a small amount of stress is transferred to you. It may be important that counselor's selfless actions be understood through the perspective of secondary stress experienced during counseling. In using a metaphor to make this point, if stress was water in a glass, practicing selfless acts in counseling would be manageable until the water reaches the rim of the glass.

In the story regarding Janet, she slowly accumulated secondhand stress by the overload of clients. She stayed successful until the water reached the rim of the glass. At that point, her beliefs and her view of the profession began to shift. Putting this in perspective, let us assess how stress operates in one's experiences. There seem to be similarities between a few large stressors affecting you and many small stressors affecting your ability to cope with stress. For example, post-traumatic stress disorder and overexposure to secondhand stress may have similar outcomes. One presents with large stressors while the other shows through a series of small ones. However, stress is stress, and how you fill the glass with stress with large traumas or a series of small ones may be less important than how full the glass becomes.

Overuse of Compassion

One of the dangers of overusing selfless acts as a counselor is that it may lead to your own trauma and stress. From personal experience, I have seen counselors hold back when they had the opportunity to practice selfless acts with clients only to see clients back away and not trust the counseling process. Conversely, I have seen highly successful counselors practice selfless acts but without knowing when to slow down, psychologically and emotionally, and, eventually, hurt themselves with their efforts. This may lead to realizing how important "knowing your limit" can be when practicing selfless acts. Compassion, generosity, and other forms of altruistic behavior while counseling others sometimes leads to being too responsible—which is itself irresponsible.

Emotional Exhaustion

When physically exhausted, one of the most important activities is sleep. When emotionally exhausted, one of the worst activities is sleep. When practicing selfless acts in counseling, it may be important to consider actions from a whole-person viewpoint. If you are going to collect secondary stress from clients continuously, it may be wise to develop activities that can counteract the emotional exhaustion that may be connected to secondary stress. Exercise, mindfulness, and other forms of self-maintenance allow your mind to seek out a restful state.

Confusion over Beliefs

Here is where experiential counselors begin to get in trouble with stress. What they believe while practicing selfless acts, and what they feel when experiencing too much stress, can create trauma within the counselor going through this pattern. It seems confusing to believe in helping clients yet at the same time feeling overcome with stress. At the risk of oversimplifying this experience, let us describe it neurologically. On the one hand, you have the dorsomedial prefrontal cortex intently wanting to be a part of selfless activity while the exhausted nervous system instructs our body to release stress hormones, including adrenaline, noradrenaline, and cortisol (Blake 2017). Under these conditions, can a counselor's beliefs win out over her or his nervous system when the body is stressed? For many in this circumstance, the answer may be no. Counselors have seen in therapy how some clients have lost a sense of their beliefs while going through, for example, a disorder based on anxiety or depression. This also may hold true for the counselor going through compassion fatigue.

Secondary Traumatic Stress Disorder

Some counselors may experience what has been called secondary traumatic stress disorder (STSD), which presents with similar symptoms as post-traumatic stress disorder (Figley 2002; Stahl and Goldstein 2010). Angry outbursts, hypervigilance, cynicism, emotional exhaustion, and exaggerated startle response are symptomatic of STSD. However, it is only recently that you will find STSD presented in the *DSM-5*. Counselors may feel a connection to clients who have experienced disasters or tragic deaths, but with no biological markers being presented, the *DSM-5* has reluctantly decided to include this phenomenon. Nevertheless, caregivers can become victimized by the secondhand trauma associated with their commitment to caring for others (Ladd and Churchill 2012).

From this description of STSD, it appears that selfless acts in therapy are a risky business. When looking at the phenomenon of selfless acts, altruism, positive regard, and other attempts at caring for clients, it does appear risky. Any emotional connection has its risks. However, with risk comes the reward of helping clients grow and change. Selfless acts appear to be a part of what is practiced by experiential talk therapists. Yet, selfless acts have their limits, and so it becomes important that counselors also know their limitations. In the end, selfless acts seem to be beneficial when both the client and counselor experience a sense of equity in the experience. Under these circumstances, an overuse of selfless acts can throw equity out of balance.

PHENOMENOLOGY AND SELFLESS ACTION

It was years since Dorian had contacted his mentor from the mental health clinic, and it was a complete surprise running into him at the movie theater. After making initial greetings, Dorian began to talk about some of his mentor's old clients and how they were doing. For the most part, they were doing well, and many had successfully moved on in their lives. However, the one thing all of them mentioned was to ask how his mentor was doing. There were many that still honored and respected him, and Dorian asked his mentor if he could tell him about one of them.

Dorian began; there is this elderly woman who is now living in a home for the aging. She is a religious woman, and every night before she goes to bed, she thanks people for giving her a long and prosperous life. I was asked to visit her by the administration at the home for the aging, who said that she had fond memories many years ago while going to you for counseling at the clinic. Every evening before she goes to bed, she prays and thanks certain relatives in her prayers. Over the months, I have stayed with her long enough to hear her prayers. At the end of her prayers each night, she makes a special effort to thank you. I do not know what your experience was with this woman, but she certainly holds you in high regard.

Dorian's mentor replied that he had done very little because the client helped herself, but they did have a close relationship long after the end of counseling. The mentor did say that one year at Christmas he gave her a Hudson Bay jacket that she seemed to wear every time he would see her. At the time, it did not appear to be a big deal, even though he knew she was alone and poor. Dorian said to his mentor that he believed that it was a bigger deal than he could imagine. Dorian stated that the lesson he learned from counseling is that people do not forget you if they sense you care about them. I believe that clients would like counselors to help them succeed in dealing with their problems, but maybe more importantly, they appreciate when you try and truly care. Regardless of whether it is in a therapy session or just an acknowledgment at some future date when counseling has long been forgotten—they may not forget you as a person.

In this story, we see that selfless acts at some point may stop being a counseling issue and may turn into a human issue where an act of compassion is not evaluated as a counseling technique but something more from the heart. Such acts are difficult to break down phenomenologically, but let us attempt to do just that, knowing that only a portion of such acts can be captured in words. In understanding selfless actions, let us now map out these interactions and why they may add to success in the therapy process. Here is a phenomenological essential pattern that a client may go through while experiencing selfless actions.[2]

Selfless Actions

Reach outside Yourself

People have a positive record of reaching out in a selfless manner when others are in severe trouble. Through hurricanes, mass shootings, and other catastrophes, people come forth to help others when it is obvious that they need help. As stated earlier in this chapter, research has found that the response from the dorsomedial prefrontal cortex in people's minds predicted subsequent altruistic behavior based on when a situation is equitable. Under these circumstances, people tend to be unselfish (Waytz, Zaki, and Mitchell 2012). The reason being that both the victims of disaster and those who help them find themselves in an equitable set of circumstances—it only seems fair to help someone in need.

Reaching out as a counselor would then appear to be a common experience in counseling when clients are seeking your help. Reaching out may be one of the important initial responses from counselors when clients enter counseling. Fortunately, in the middle of a disaster, victims are not required to fill out forms based on family history, past symptomatic behavior, and other procedures before reaching out to someone. Yet, traditional medical model procedures might want to reconsider when to reach out as a professional and when to reach out as a human being. From a more phenomenological approach, institutional procedures found in the counseling experience may need to be separated in some way from dealing with client problems. Client crisis can outweigh counselor procedures. It may be the first encounter with a client where the tone in counseling is set for the subsequent counseling sessions.

Find Meaning in Others

"The more one forgets himself—by giving himself to a cause to serve or another person to love—the more human he is," said Viktor E. Frankl (2011). Finding one's humanity in life can be sought after from many different perspectives. For talk therapists, it is finding meaning in one's self to help others that allows you to find meaning in the client—so that meaning benefits both parties. When counselors find meaning in the pain experienced by clients, selfless acts of compassion, empathy, and positive regard begin to flow more freely in the dialogue created between them. It is the integration of two separate minds coming together where selfless acts can contribute to the healing process (Fosha, Siegel, and Solomon 2009).

Actively Listen

One of the powerful methods for practicing selfless acts with clients is to listen actively. This process demonstrates that the counselor is willing to put their thoughts and behavior aside to find meaning in the client's thoughts and feelings. Active listening, beyond being a method for understanding the meaning behind a client's experiences, is also a selfless act of compassion.

For example, a client stormed into the counselor's office yelling, crying, and accusing the counselor of doing very little to take away the pain of her husband's recent death. The counselor's response was to actively listen as the client attacked him. For over a half an hour, the attack went on as the counselor selflessly allowed it to happen without any form of retaliation. In the end, the client apologized for the outburst but said that she needed to attack someone. The counselor responded, "Then I am glad you picked me."

Immersed in the Client's Experience

This example demonstrates how deeply a more experiential mental health counselor helps a client in crisis. Sometimes it takes more courage than intellect to be an effective experientially oriented counselor. However, immersing yourself in client problems is different than identifying with them or owning them. Counselors are responsible "to" clients not "for" them, and crisis is no time to be relating to a client's pain with one's own pain. What is important is to immerse one's self into the client's pain so that the client comes to the realization that you understand it and are a part of it (van den Berg 1972). Selfless acts of this nature sometimes take courage to go where the client is at. The outside world may view a completely different perception taking place when a counselor enters the world of the client. For example, for the outside world, attacking a counselor for the recent death of a loved one could be taken as inappropriate and disturbing, yet by the counselor immersing himself or herself into the client's world, it is a part of humanity's ongoing dialogue where the entire incident makes sense.

Deeper Human Connection

It seems redundant at this point to continue coming back to the importance of the dialogue between client and counselor, but selfless acts are a part of that dialogue. Positive regard, empathy, intuition, attunement, insight, and selfless acts make up the foundation of this dialogue, so they are important to experiential talk therapists. This type of counseling considers client behaviors, thoughts, and emotions but is also concerned with meaning at a deeper level of connection. For this type of counseling, the whole person experience of the client is considered, not just symptoms. It may be more important to understand who you are as a person than what symptoms keep haunting you.

Neurologically, it may be important to reconsider the integrated mind when talking about deeper human connections. Mind emerges out of energy and information that flows through our interpersonal connections, our brain, and whole body (embodied brain), where this energy and information self-organizes all at once and in all directions (Siegel 2016). From a phenomenological viewpoint, deeper human connections help to organize the mind in an integrated manner so more meaningful dialogue can emerge. Selfless acts help in this integration by opening the pathway for deeper human connections between client and counselor. Selfless acts are more than altruistic behavior in phenomenological talk therapy. They are a commitment to "being with" a client, wherever that path may take them.

DISCUSSION

The most answered comment when asked, "Why do you want to be a mental health counselor?" after personally interviewing hundreds of candidates for graduate school is, "I want to help people." Such a belief on its surface seems generalized and a bit abstract. From a phenomenological, experiential perspective, it is vital that such statements be operationalized into something more concrete and more usable. From my perspective, experiential talk therapists need a better understanding of specific phenomenological experiences before they delve into the experiences of others.

Selfless acts are one of those experiences. Studying concrete procedures and techniques in talk therapy have their place in understanding and helping clients. Such issues as cognitive behavioral therapy, behavioral therapy, acceptance and commitment therapy, mindfulness, person-centered therapy, dialectical behavioral therapy, and many others have their place in the education of new talk therapists, along with understanding the *DSM-5*, and symptoms that go with each disorder. However, embedded in all of us are certain characteristics that make us human. Some of the characteristics presented in this book have demonstrated more human characteristics, such as insight, intuition, empathy, and attunement. These also are important to learn for those therapists pursuing a career in talk therapy. Selfless acts take their place along with these other human characteristics that show therapists as human beings and not only as experts in the field of human conflict.

NOTES

1. It is accurate to point out that we do have neurological mechanisms to protect us from danger. The hypothalamus area of the brain, and especially the amygdala, is designed as one of our "crisis centers." When danger is prevalent, there is no reason to only rely on the cerebral cortex to process a logical solution to a crisis. The middle brain can process this information much more quickly and respond more effectively to crisis. Therefore, in some ways, we are wired to be vigilant, cautious, and reactive. However, this does not negate the power of selfless acts and the meaning they bring to our lives. Ladd, Peter. 2017. "Why Emotional Addictions Rob You of Feeling Fully Human: Implications for Addictions & Mental Health Counseling," *New York State Psychological Association Annual Conference,* June 2, 2017.

2. Trying to describe selfless acts can be problematic. Much of what makes up this phenomenon goes beyond the written word. The essence of selfless acts may be as much a visual experience as a written one. Some phenomena are better expressed in images. Selfless acts may be more a visual expression when trying to capture this phenomenon than what can be described through words. For more information on this subject matter, refer to the following: Benedek, András, and Kristóf Nyíri. 2014. *The Power of the Image: Emotion, Expression, and Explanation.* New York, NY, Peter Lang GmbH, Internationaler Verlag der Wissenschaften .

Chapter Eight

Fear

Positive or Negative?

NEUROSCIENCE AND FEAR

In therapy, fearful clients may have to take into consideration neurological, physiological, anatomic, and cognitive factors. Fearful behavior affects specific areas of the client's brain and central nervous system, hormonal secretions, and arousal; basically, the entire physiological system of the body is affected (Bocanegra and Zeelenberg 2011). Fear is said to affect muscle tension, respiration rate, cardiac output, blood sugar level, salivary output, blood pressure, and so on. Neurologically, the amygdala, brainstem, diencephalon, or insular cortex senses the body's most primal inner signals of danger when basic survival is threatened (De Groot, Smeets, and Semin 2015). Regarding the amygdala, much of the fear we perceive from the outside world is filtered through the limbic area, which is where the amygdala resides. Specifically, fear is a complex process that is still not entirely understood though certain responses to fear are commonly perceived in everyday living. The common responses to being afraid are to fight, flight, or freeze.

In therapy, we see clients in all three of these modalities: the client who feels enraged while they feel the emotion of fear underneath; the client who wants to run away from those fearful circumstances that cause feelings of fear; and the client frozen with fear who is unable to talk or behave rationally. It is our responsibility as talk therapists to help clients confront these fears with a form of action to help normalize their fearful reaction. Confronting a fear instead of backing down from it can bring about a sense of accomplishment and empowerment. When you confront your fear, you have a higher possibility of gaining personal power. Every time you confront your fear, you accumulate evidence of your ability to cope—a feeling of "I did it once. I can do it again" (Shpancer 2010).

In therapy, fear can be a positive experience. For example, fear is a fundamental part of making responsive decisions. The amygdala is an important source of feeling that something is emotionally wrong or isn't quite right. By reminding us of potential risk and harm, this primitive center can put the brakes on other impulses. Even though some people let fear get in the way of long-term goals, it may be a mistake to think the solution is to overcome all fear (McGonigal 2010).

From a phenomenological perspective, it is important for a client to understand both positive and negative aspects of fear. Such an understanding may help the counselor to apply different techniques to modulating, eliminating, or just learning from fear. For example, neurologically, the amygdala may help in making quick decisions long before our brain's emotional and logical center, the pre-frontal cortex, has a chance to assess any given situation (Adolphs, Tranel, Damasio, and Damasio 1995). For the talk therapist, it may be important that clients understand not only a neurological perspective regarding fear but also a phenomenological perspective. Here is a story to make this point.

Fear was a constant worry for Mary as she entered the counselor's office. It seemed her fear encompassed many different facets of her life. She was afraid of meeting new people, afraid of failure, afraid of speaking in public, and afraid that she was going to die. Peter, her counselor, wanted her to talk about these fears, to get them out on the table so she could look at them and understand them. Much of Mary's venting about her fears seemed to depict that being afraid would be her ultimate demise. She spoke about it as though it was out there in the world and it could attack her at any time under the right conditions.

Peter decided to educate Mary about how fear works. He said that with some fears you will experience something affecting you from the world. For example, suddenly someone might ask her to speak in public, or she might feel fear of driving a car in busy traffic. Other fears are more within you, such as fear of failure or fear of death, and others are somewhere in the middle, such as fear of meeting new people. The first thing that Peter wanted to share is that fear can be positive or negative based on how it is used during each day. This was the first revelation for Mary who had previously perceived it as a phenomenon unto itself and did not realize that she had a part in how it works. Peter also went into how fear is processed neurologically. He explained that in traumatic situations the amygdala sends a signal that causes fear while at other times it is the amygdala that guards us against making foolish mistakes, such as stepping out into traffic or avoiding an alley that looks dangerous. He also said that fear could be a negative force in her life when it freezes her or bottles her up.

Mary understood that her vague, generalized version of fear probably added to her problem. Changing the meaning behind fear was the first step in clarifying how she would face fear in the future. Peter asked what fear she wanted to work on first. Which is the one that means the most to her? She candidly admitted that her fear of death was the one that haunted her the most. After a few sessions, Peter had an insight that all her other fears were based on a fear of life, not of death, such as meeting new people, fear of speaking in public, and fear of failure. What is it about life that Mary is afraid to face? That was the question Mary left with as the session ended that day.

At the next session, Mary told Peter that his insight made sense and asked him how did he figure that out? Peter said that he had no idea, but the statement "being afraid of life" seemed to be building between them and kept pointing in that direction, so he just said it. Mary responded by saying, "You are correct, I am afraid to live. I have spent most of my time being afraid of many things, and time will eventually run out for me if I keep thinking about death." Peter said to Mary, "Do you remember when I told you the amygdala in our brains can protect us from danger or it can be used to fight, flight, or freeze? Maybe your issue is not getting rid of your fear but learning how to use it in a productive manner." From this point, specific techniques were used to work through the fears; some of them included mindfulness and exposure therapy. When Mary had a breakthrough with each one of them, Peter would go back to the issue of being afraid of life and assess how these accomplishments were affecting her longstanding fear of death. With each accomplishment, fear of death slowly became a moot point and life began to hold more meaning for Mary.

From a neurological perspective, Mary's amygdala shifted from a negative perspective where cortisol and adrenaline were consistently being aroused depending on the level of fear, to switching to neurons called GABA (gamma-Aminobutyric acid) that helped to sooth Mary as she worked through her fear of life.[1] From a phenomenological perspective, the basic structure of the experience was discussed with her, only to find out that Mary had a vague and confusing understanding regarding her fear of death but found meaning in her fear of life—of wasting time as she grew older. Neurologically, Mary learned something from her connections with Peter. She was educated in how fear can be either a positive or a negative depending on how you look at it. Phenomenologically, Peter learned that by keeping an open mind and staying attuned to Mary's story, what emerged was an understanding that Mary had a bigger fear of life than of death. This would probably not happen if she was given a diagnosis based on symptoms and followed a strict medical model treatment plan. However, the dialogue between them revealed prophetic information that transformed therapy into a meaningful, educational experience.

PHENOMENOLOGY AND FEAR

Looking at this story from a medical model perspective may have drawn different conclusions than those adopted by Peter. A diagnosis may have been made that Mary had a form of social anxiety disorder to counteract her fear of meeting people and needed some cognitive behavioral therapy or possibly medication. The diagnosis could have been based on some phobias such as a fear of public speaking where a form of exposure therapy may have been prescribed for her. Her fear of failure may have been faced with solution-based brief therapy regarding the positive accomplishments in her life. All these could have helped her. However, they all were based on the symptoms she was presenting and not on where she was at as a whole person in her life. How the counselor perceived Mary obviously was important. Peter perceived her as someone who was afraid of life but not necessarily afraid of death. However, that perception was not based on her symptoms but on the many angles found in the dialogue between them while building a therapeutic alliance. It was a perception based on insight, not incremental building of a case for a specific disorder.

Another point to make is that Mary, when entering Peter's office, may not have been presenting any specific fear at all. Much of what she discussed was her anxiety about specific situations and events. Even her fear of death was generalized, and in the end, not accurate, which was part of the problem facing Mary. She was identifying herself as a fearful person not as a person going through anxiety. It was only after she had an insightful moment between sessions that her most accurate problem was revealed to her. In this form of counseling, the process follows the person, not the symptoms. Mary, as a person, had found a purpose and meaning in her life, and it was to live it as best she could. It was her distorted fear of death that clouded the water for any substantive growth and change.

With a change in Mary as a person, other behavioral changes became more viable. Cognitive behavioral therapy made sense in helping her with fear of socializing. Emersion in some form of exposure therapy may now make sense if she wants to overcome a fear of public speaking. Or, maybe her fear of facing possible failure has become irrelevant now that fear has been clarified for her. She knows that failure is based on living, not dying. In these, Mary can grow and change, yet it may be that clarifying the threat based on a fear of living allowed her to take a stand and to risk and to find purpose and meaning in her life.

PHENOMENOLOGY AND ANXIETY

As much as it is important to separate negative fear from fear that is beneficial, it may be as important to separate the phenomenon of anxiety from fear. One quick definition of the difference may be surmised that anxiety is fear of the unknown; though, for most practical purposes, that does not really give us much to go on. However, they are neurologically and phenomenologically connected to each other. The terms fear and anxiety sometimes have been interchangeable; however, in counseling, they should not be used in that manner. Fear describes feelings that occur when the source of harm, the threat, is either immediate or imminent as in having an angry dog chase you down the street or if someone has told you that a bully is seeking to beat you up. Anxiety describes feelings that occur when the source of harm is uncertain or at a distance in space or time, such as, for example, in a vague sense of being afraid to die (LeDoux and Pine 2016).

Neurologically, let us look at two different systems regarding how fear and anxiety work, and then separate fear from anxiety. Fear is often said to be an innate function of subcortical brain areas. This view stems from the idea that humans inherited certain basic, universally expressed emotions often described as products of the brain's limbic system. It is in the limbic area that the amygdala resides, which is frequently said to be a "fear center," or, in more contemporary terminology, the hub of a "fear circuit" (LeDoux and Pine 2016). This system can be beneficial and serves to protect us from harm. However, another system includes the ventromedial prefrontal cortex in responding to fear and anxiety, which means that we can consciously control fear or anxiety through our thinking and perceptions (LeDoux 2012). With fear, that usually means that we are aware of the threat and are clear as to why it is threatening and have time to take a stand on how to respond to it. With anxiety, it usually means that we are not completely aware of the threat and hold a level of uncertainty about if/when the threat will harm us.

For the phenomenological-oriented counselor, this means that sometimes clients are startled by a fearful event where their crisis centers take over and work to protect them from the fearful situation. Other times, the ventromedial prefrontal cortex of a client's brain has something to say in how a client perceives and responds to fear. For example, in the story about Mary, she responded with anxiety when she thought about and perceived an imagined threat about her death. However, when the threat was clarified, she was not faced with anxiety but fear of doing something about her perceived purposeless life.

In my experience, I have observed some clients believing that if they could get through their anxiety, then they may achieve happiness, normality, stability, and so forth. Sometimes, the shock comes when they have clarified the threat to their problems only to find that now they are afraid. Fortunately, in this situation, fear may be the way out of their pain. Now they can take a stand on facing their problems by working through their fear to solve them. With anxiety, no stand seems clarified, and no future problem-solving seems imminent.[2]

Pattern of Anxiety

When we compare anxiety with fear from a phenomenological point of view, the essence of each phenomenon appears different in human experience (Ladd and Blanchfield 2016). Such a clarification is based on differences and the similarities between these two phenomena. First, it is impossible to get through life without a certain level of anxiety. Too much anxiety and one may develop an anxiety disorder; too little anxiety, and it may thwart one's purpose in life for trying new experiences. A moderate amount of anxiety is needed to stay alert in an ever-changing world. From a medical model perspective, there is a spectrum of disorders where anxiety is attached to them. Post-traumatic stress disorder (PTSD), obsessive-compulsive disorder (OCD), generalized anxiety disorder (GAD), and attention-deficit disorder (ADD) are just a few. So, in the scope of mental health counseling, anxiety is something both client and counselors may have to face together.

Uncertainty

Most of us live with uncertainty every day and still manage to find purpose and meaning in the world. Any attempt to rid ourselves of all uncertainty seems an unreasonable request. It may be a certain amount of uncertainty helps us learn new experiences in our lives by changing uncertainty to certainty. However, for all of us, it would make sense to not perceive uncertainty as something negative even when having stressful experiences. If we avoid most of the uncertainty in our lives, we avoid life. From a phenomenological perspective, uncertainty can lead to a major problem, or one can see it as a starting point for growth and change.

The role of the phenomenologically oriented counselor is to give clients an opportunity to talk about their uncertainty. Whether an answer is found to relieve it may not be the most important aspect of discussing one's uncertainty with a counselor. In collaboration with a counselor, the client understands the uncertain aspects of living beginning to take shape. The counselor helps develop certain boundaries that a client can look at their uncertainty from different perspectives within the safety of the counseling process. The goal may be to put anxiety into perspective as to what is reasonable. In collaborating with a counselor, the client's understanding of uncertain aspects of living take shape, and experiencing anxiety is one of them.

Focus Narrows

Sometimes clients seek counseling because their methods of dealing with uncertainty have become overwhelming. When clients try to solve personal problems and get nowhere, they can stop focusing on other portions of their lives. For example, trying to deal with uncertainty after losing your job may have you thinking about the job loss most of the time. When your focus narrows, such as while thinking about the loss of the job, you are not thinking of other things that may bring you pleasure or give you confidence. This can feel overwhelming. You may be narrowing your focus to solve the problem of job loss but what happens if there are no answers available at that time? Anxiety begins to form when one keeps thinking about a life problem and forgets to think about those positive things that expand one's focus and give confidence. There seems to be nothing wrong with narrowing your focus to solve a problem, but if you cannot then expand it, one slowly can become overwhelmed and may experience anxiety.

Constant Rumination

Unable to expand one's focus can lead to constant worry or rumination. Neurologically and metaphorically, this may mean the switch on your amygdala is broken. Constant rumination encourages the release of cortisol based on the threat found in the anxious client (Simsek 2017). Uncertainty leads to a narrow focus, which leads to not being able to expand one's focus, further leading to constant rumination where neurologically and experientially a client's sense of control may begin to fade.

For example, a client comes to counseling and says, "I do not know what is wrong with me. I cannot stop thinking about why she left, and I am starting to feel out of control." Constant worry or rumination begins to change the neurological makeup within the embodied brain (brain and body), how a person organizes their information and energy regarding how they think, and the difficulty this new combination affects interpersonal relationships. In other words, the client finds it difficult to calm down because he or she is thinking too much, which lays the groundwork for feeling out of control.

Symptoms Develop

Symptoms are where one will find most of the information found in the *DSM* regarding some form of anxiety. From a medical model, these symptoms are the primary focus of medical model counselors dealing with an anxious client. From a phenomenological model, these symptoms are only a part of understanding the whole person's anxiety. Uncertainty, a narrow focus, not being able to expand one's focus, and constant rumination are all considered a part of the anxiety experience from a phenomenological perspective. At this point, from a medical model, much of the treatment now focuses on symptoms reduction and symptoms maintenance. From a pharmaceutically based medical model, the focus now becomes how are we as professionals neurologically going to administer the correct remedy by using psychotropic drugs and a bona fide treatment plan.

Crisis Mode

As stated earlier in this book, a medical model seems to be most effective in dealing with a crisis, so the formula of psychotropic drugs and some counseling technique tends to make sense. However, from a phenomenological model, what happens to all other facets of the anxiety experience? After the client has been stabilized, is there any remedy that treats the whole person, or gives meaning to the anxiety experience? Forming a therapeutic alliance with the client allows these issues to emerge without needing a treatment plan and to insightfully emerge through meaningful dialogue that clarifies how the anxiety makes sense in the client's world.

PATTERN OF FEAR FOUND IN COUNSELING

So far, this chapter has discussed fear from a neurological and phenomenological perspective, pointing out differences and similarities between anxiety and fear. Also, an attempt was made to separate imminent experiences with fear, such as being mugged by a criminal, to more long-standing experiences, such as being threatened by a bully who you may run into later in the day. This part of the chapter focuses on how fear is experienced during counseling sessions and how it may be a beneficial step toward recovery. In a more generalized description of fear during counseling, it can appear as a disorder, such as a phobia, or a threat that needs some form of extinction, or as a life experience that needs some form of modulation, such as a fear of being criticized by loved ones. The following pattern looks at fear differently. It depicts how fear can be a major process in the counseling experience and how avoiding it may make whatever counseling problem a client is experiencing even worse.

Pattern of Fear

Feeling Threatened

Steve had a difficult problem to consider. He had been working with Kyle, a mental health counselor, regarding the presenting problem of anxiety after Steve's family walked out on him six months ago. When entering counseling, he was in such disarray that Kyle asked him to see a psychiatrist who prescribed antianxiety medicine when his anxiety would reach critical mass. The rest of the time was spent with Kyle working through what went wrong in the marriage. During these six months, different issues emerged, such as guilt, communication problems, the resentment displayed by his wife, and how Steve felt by letting down his children. These were all meaningful issues that needed to be discussed and worked through, and Steve had done an adequate job working through them with the help Kyle gave him. However, now Steve felt threatened. He assumed that once he worked through his problems that he would be free to start his life over again. When Kyle asked him how he now felt, Steve's response was the emotion of fear.

The assumption made by Steve was that once he worked through his problems, he would be free to move on. This is made by many clients who enter counseling. Their hope with counseling can be the same hope they may expect when taking psychotropic drugs; namely, if I take these drugs, then I will be relieved of my suffering. In many cases, these assumptions are incorrect. For example, the successful work accomplished by Kyle and Steve in counseling presented a new issue for Steve. Steve felt threatened with what he may be doing next in his life. The question that may arise in Steve's mind is, "How much have I really accomplished in counseling if I now feel threatened about my future?" The answer to that question is yes and that he has accomplished a great deal. Before counseling, he was drowning himself with anxiety about his present life, but now that was over. He was now clear on what happened to him. His new threat was what to do about it.

Clarifying the Threat

Once a client finds out about the basic meaning behind their problem, for example, Steve becoming aware of the nature of his anxiety, then the focus of counseling can shift from being aware of the problem to what are you going to do about it. In the case of Steve, there was a shift away from being anxious to a sense of fear. After an actual threat is clarified with clients, they now are in a position to take a stand. In some respects, fear forces people to choose where they stand on a threat. For example, after Steve clarified the source of his fear, he now was faced with the choice of either being satisfied with awareness of his presenting problems or to do something about them for the future.

Taking a Stand

Many clients go through counseling and are aware of the suffering and pain they have experienced, but when asked, "What do you want to do about it?" they feel threatened with fear. Sometimes growth and change require more than clarifying threats. It also may require some form of action to take place. In cases of anxiety, some clients do not want to continue because they believe their anxiety is returning when they are put in the position of taking a stand with their lives. For the most part, in this position, they are not experiencing a return to anxiety but the fear that accompanies new growth and change.

The fear that may go along with taking a stand with client problems can be therapeutic. For example, one of the main problems with anxiety is the inability to take a stand because the threat has yet to be clarified. With the threat clarified, taking a stand may require working through one's fear. Passively, to be aware of problems in counseling may not be enough to overcome them. Fear may be the great motivator or the great discourager when a client arrives at that moment when it seems time to take a stand on his or her counseling problems.

Go into Action

This is where action-based therapies can be helpful in client's working through their fear of growth and change.[3] In a phenomenological approach to counseling, there is a time to develop a therapeutic alliance, a time to identify a problem, and a time for action. As I have said throughout this book, premature action plans run the risk of coming up with highly effective treatment but possibly connected to the wrong problems. For example, developing an action plan around only clearing up Steve's family problems from a phenomenological perspective does not go far enough in establishing a whole person experience in Steve's life. Without dealing with Steve's fear of the future, he now has awareness about his past experiences but no plan for his future experiences.

Resilience

Facing one's fears, taking a stand, and going into action can create a sense of resilience in fearful clients. Eliminating all client fears may be counterproductive when one considers how working through future fears can create a sense of resilience. Over the years, I have seen, for example, a medical model use of psychotropic drugs to eliminate or at least modify client fears of the future. In the administration of these drugs, the symptom of fear has been successfully reduced or eliminated. However, fear reduction, without considering how working through fear can be beneficial for future experiences, seems to be solving one problem by creating another. Coping with one's fears is quite different than growing and changing by working through them. In using a metaphor, the choice may be waiting for the next shoe to drop as opposed to being prepared for when it drops. Fear may be one of many avenues to developing resilience in clients, and an overgeneralization of fear in counseling seems to do no one any good. The medical model's approach to fear reduction or elimination is closely associated with their approach to anxiety. Reduce the symptoms to solve the problem. In a phenomenological model, finding meaning in how clients experience fear adds a more accurate perspective when working with fearful clients.

DISCUSSION

Fear may be a bit different than other emotions clients experience in their lives, based on research that can specifically, link fear to the amygdala portion of our brains (Gonzalez 2011). In other words, fear is the exclusive emotion of the amygdala and, as such, controls many different biological and experiential processes in human beings. This chapter pointed out a few of them but most specifically how fear can be used in the counseling process as a partial motivator for growth and change. Someone asked me a while back whether in combat a soldier is better off being afraid or not being afraid, regarding personal survival. I quoted him a statement heard or read (I cannot remember its source), but it made sense to me: "Fear can stop you from being stupid, so I think it has its place in combat."

I believe that the phenomenon of fear has its place in counseling and therapy and not just as a symptom of a disorder or a disorder itself. Fear in counseling may be somewhere between using common sense and not being stupid about it—and using it as a counseling technique. Being afraid to work through life's problems is just that—a life problem. Feeling more balanced after counseling may not be possible without working through some aspect of being afraid. Working through fear can be an act of resilience. It can be the suffering one needs to experience before one can feel a sense of meaningful intentionality in one's life.

NOTES

1. Studies have shown that GABA is a support for the digestive tract, improving bowel function, epithelial regeneration, better muscle mass, and a more restful sleep. It has also been observed that such supplementation has a lower susceptibility to stress and produces greater concentration and work efficiency. Such activity is extremely beneficial for physically active people. Abdou, Adham, S. Higashiqchi, Kim Horie, M. Kim, and H. Yokogoshi. 2006. "Relaxation and Immunity Enhancement Effects of Gamma-Aminobutyric Acid (GABA) Administration in Humans." *Biofactors* 26, no. 3: 201–8.

2. Working through one's fears in counseling may be more difficult than taking psychotropic drugs to reduce one's fear. The difference may be that working through fear can create resilience and give a client confidence when the next fear arises. The choice goes back to the medical model of wanting to get rid of all suffering and not seeing the value in necessary suffering that goes along with working through one's fears. Ladd, Peter. 2009. *Emotional Addictions: A Reference Book for mental Health and Addictions Counselors*. Lanham, MD: University Press of America.

3. Action-based counseling techniques, such as cognitive behavioral therapy, dialectical behavioral therapy, mindfulness therapy, and acceptance and commitment therapy, are a good fit for this stage of working through one's fears. When starting these therapies too early, the

groundwork for taking a stand may be premature. Beliefs lead to behavior, and in this stage of taking a stand, action behavior makes more sense. Ladd, Peter D. and AnnMarie Churchill. 2012. *Person-Centered Diagnosis and Treatment in Mental Health: A Model for Empowering Clients.* London, UK: Jessica Kingsley Publishing, 1–25.

Chapter Nine

Momentum

MOMENTUM IN COUNSELING

The phenomenon of momentum is referred in the field of mental health as psychological momentum (Iso-Ahola and Mobily 1980). Much of the literature is in the field of athletics where studies have been done on how this phenomenon plays a part in athletic events.[1] What follows is an example from athletics. While watching a boxing event, I observed the change in momentum happening three times. The boxers were of equal size, skill level, and overall competence. The first time the momentum changed was when boxer 1 knocked down boxer 2 in the fourth round. The momentum changed again in the sixth round when boxer 2 knocked down boxer 1. It looked like, at this point, the fight was over based on the condition of boxer 1. Suddenly, in the eleventh round, boxer 1 gained momentum and knocked out boxer 2, which ended the fight. All involved in the fight declared that it was momentum that determined the outcome.

In counseling clients, the phenomenon of momentum seems lost among psychotropic drugs, counseling techniques, and treatment plans. However, in my experience, momentum plays an important part not only in client recovery but also in how a client becomes addicted or possesses a mental health disorder. Here are a few analogies that I have heard regarding momentum: Counseling is like rolling a snowball down a hill. At first, you need to push it, but at a certain point, it is big enough that it moves on its own momentum. Here is another analogy: A person can say they have an addiction, but at a certain point, the addiction has them. Whether we are talking about playing with snowballs or mapping out a path of an addiction, both consider momentum as a major part of each experience. Like a forest fire, momentum can gain energy based on its own momentum, and so can the experience of talk therapy.

Psychological momentum is defined as an added or gained psychological power that changes interpersonal perceptions and influences an individual's mental performance (Iso-Ahola and Dotson 2016). Research suggests that the main psychological processes that underpin momentum effects are confidence, perceived competence, and intrinsic motivation (Rosenqvist and Skans 2015). Based on related research, it is hypothesized that momentum starts as a conscious process but subsequently becomes a major facilitator of nonconscious automatic execution of human behavior and performance (Hubbard 2015).

One of the first observations is that momentum in counseling has to do with empowerment. Not initially when client and counselor are getting to know each other but after a meaningful dialogue is formed in the client and counselor relationship. In many respects, relationships, in general, are based partially on momentum. As the dialogue grows, people may go from consciously establishing the relationship to unconsciously allowing momentum to move it along at its own pace. This may happen based on the fact that at the beginning of a relationship both parties are figuring out some unspoken rules for the relationship to continue. Later, when the relationship is formed, little conscious effort needs to go into consciously playing by these relationship rules. For example, is the relationship between client and counselor going to be formal or informal? Is the client going to practice a treatment plan devised by the counselor, or is the client free to seek out her or his personal journey while interacting with the counselor?

Research shows that confidence is a major ingredient that adds to momentum (Iso-Ahola and Dotson 2016). In talk therapy, confidence is one of the reasons for creating a meaningful dialogue—either confidence in one's self as a client or confidence in the therapist to keep the momentum moving. By creating a meaningful dialogue, both parties consciously build confidence and trust, but they also start the possibility for momentum to kick in at any moment and at any time. In more medical model talk therapy, momentum is not as big an issue. Performing tasks designated by a treatment plan are more of a step-by-step approach to counseling where momentum hopefully happens in the action phase where techniques are being tried through practice.

Empathy and selfless acts by the therapist can also build momentum. Both characteristics help with the client's perceived competence. Clients may come to counseling with an extraordinarily low level of perceived competence. However, by the counselor practicing empathy and expressing acts of positive regard, momentum begins to grow in the client. For example, some clients enter counseling with negative momentum. They may be so hard on themselves that it may take establishing a meaningful dialogue to turn momentum around and go in a more positive direction. One of my observations in a medical model treatment plan has been to see treatment start while the client still has negative momentum. If you believe momentum is important, it will make sense to stop the negative momentum and begin to build a more positive momentum before any serious intervention takes place.

Another aspect of momentum is found in the importance of intrinsic motivation in counseling (Hunt, Rietschel, Hatfield, and Iso-Ahola 2013). I have believed for some years that clients want to heal psychologically, but their intrinsic motivation has yet to be discovered by themselves or by the therapist or both. Momentum may help find the motivation inside. It becomes an identity issue of what one is made of and goes beyond having confidence, feeling empowered, and believing in yourself through perceived competence. Momentum is a whole person issue, and it is stimulated by themes such as hope, insight, intuitive decisions, and attuned communication. These are skills that can wake up one's intrinsic motivation.

For example: Rebecca was sexually harassed for years. After she broke away from the harassing relationship, she had the intrinsic motivation to move on with her life. However, she had been to numerous counselors who wanted to specifically talk about the trauma and nothing else. When finding a more phenomenologically oriented counseling setting, the counselor could see in Rebecca's heart that she wanted to move on but was exhausted from the harassment experience. The counselor recognized her intrinsic motivation to move on as the problem, but instead of developing a treatment plan for Rebecca's trauma, the counselor offered her hope. When the counselor had insight, she shared it with Rebecca.

The counselor stayed closely attuned to her client while momentum began to build. What the counselor found remarkable was Rebecca appeared empowered and began to make intuitive decisions regarding her future. Rebecca decided to take down pictures of her ex, and she got rid of his clothes. From that moment on, the momentum of her counseling began to soar at an unbelievable pace. Rebecca and the counselor had found that intrinsic motivation had set off momentum in her recovery. Rebecca felt unstoppable. Treating a client for trauma is certainly acceptable in this case, yet no one is going to find momentum an issue in the DSM-5. Sometimes phenomena speak to the client and counselor beyond a disorder. The "how" to heal sometimes becomes more important than the "why" to heal.

NEUROSCIENCE AND MOMENTUM

Moods are our brain's way of creating momentum. Successfully completing counseling is not a random event. It has something to do with your mood and the type of emotions making up your mood. If you have a breakthrough in counseling, a positive mood will be partially responsible for your success. If you have a breakthrough in counseling, you may learn to expect further breakthroughs, thus creating an emotional mood for continued breakthroughs, and in this manner, moods are our brain's way of creating momentum (Forte 2017). Behavioral and neural findings suggest that one's mood can influence positive outcomes when one is in a good mood relative to when one is in a bad mood (Eldar, Rutledge, Dolan, and Niv 2015). What this means for counselors is that helping clients achieve a mood that is positive may help them with positive neural firings in the brain leading to more positive outcomes—reinforcing positive momentum. Personally, it is one reason that I find myself using humor even in dire counseling situations. Not to address the counseling problem, but instead to change the momentum in the session.

So a key to understanding momentum is to understand mood (Hubbard 2015). Many regions fundamental to mood are buried deep in the most primordial parts of the brain. Changes in moods are thought to be among the first developments in the human species. This is probably because mood has evolutionary importance. Overall, the brain seems geared towards maintaining a mildly positive frame of mind. Being in a good mood makes us more likely to seek new experiences, be creative, make plans, and adapt to changing conditions (Dehaene 2014). Many people seem to believe that shutting down their emotions and banishing their moods will make them more productive. The opposite is more accurate. Mood helps create momentum and gives direction to future experiences and future aspirations.

Most of being in a good mood can be accredited to the limbic system in the brain (Feather 1968). Without the limbic system, it would be hard to believe that any momentum could take place within our brains. Emotional centers such as the hypothalamus and amygdala within the limbic system can help create momentum when the mood is right, and the right mood may come early in counseling. Also, the insula, a small region of the cerebral cortex, may help us become aware of our moods (Suzuki 2012), and in counseling, it may create momentum early in therapy. It helps in creating a therapeutic mood, more commonly referred to as a therapeutic alliance, early in therapy that allows momentum to transfer from one counseling session to another, further allowing for an accumulation of momentum.

If a client has achieved some form of momentum from the session a week earlier, then some of that session can transfer to the present counseling session; thus momentum continues in counseling. However, what happens in medical model talk therapy is that sessions are programmed to focus on different issues each week so the momentum in counseling can be interrupted. Losing that positive flow that keeps all counseling sessions in dynamic momentum may be a detriment to healing. So focusing on a task from a treatment plan is an honest effort to help clients with their problems even though momentum may be lost. Focusing on the momentum of the counseling sessions is a more phenomenological attempt to help clients move forward with their problems.

Here's an example: Lulu was struggling with her anxiety for many years. Finally, she was talked into seeking out counseling. As she entered the mental health clinic, anxiety kept rushing through her mind. The first person she met was kind and friendly and gave her a motivational interview, which started to turn around some of her anxiety.

On the next visit, she met with a psychiatrist who went down a checklist of questions about her life, and later she found out that he was gathering information to make a diagnosis regarding her possible disorders. After that meeting, she found her anxiety becoming more acute and painful, but she had started the process and was determined to finish it. The following week she met with a counselor who told Lulu to share her story and what she believed might be the cause of her anxiety. Lulu talked about her history of growing up poor and marrying young, without thinking through what all that meant. She also shared that she had what professionals called low-grade anxiety for a long time. Her counselor sat behind her desk writing down information but never explained what was in the information, or how it was going to be used. Regarding any momentum, it seemed to be lost as she waited for next week to arrive.

Later she found out that the information was taken to a case management meeting where a treatment plan was designed between the psychiatrist, initial interviewer, and the mental health counselor. Upon her return to counseling, the counselor asked Lulu to agree and sign the following treatment plan that consisted of cognitive/behavioral therapy skills, homework assignments, and the goal of reducing her anxiety. After signing the agreement, the rest of the session was spent with the psychiatrist, who gave her .05 mg of Lorazepam for when she needed it. This was followed by her counselor giving homework assignments to practice her new counseling skills. Regarding any momentum being created, little of it was present except that Lulu's anxiety was gaining momentum.

By the sixth meeting, some of the skills were working, and Lulu began to feel modest momentum beginning again. She felt the skills were helping her, so anytime she began feeling overwhelming anxiety, she would use these skills. She shared that it was helpful, especially when her husband created conflict. Lulu had gained some momentum, and her counselor felt that Lulu now had the skills to control her anxiety and made plans for ending the sessions.

Months later, she began having anxiety attacks even though the Lorazepam did help, and the counseling skills worked some of the time. One of her friends said to Lulu, "It appears that all your anxiety is coming from your relationship with your husband because that is all you talk about." The next week she made an appointment to see a more holistic counselor. When meeting with the counselor, the first statement from the counselor was, "Tell me about yourself." Lulu began talking about different issues, such as how she always was an anxious person, she had trouble controlling her anxiety, and she had deep marital problems, at least that is what people told her. Her counselor listened and let her know that he was listening, and now and then he commented on how hard it must be to carry all that around inside. At the end of the session, Lulu felt a certain momentum and looked forward to next week.

As the weeks passed, Lulu and her counselor seemed to be becoming more casual around each other. There was an unspoken rule that Lulu could talk about what was on her mind, and her counselor would stay with her at every moment along the way. Being that attuned, the counselor had little trouble pointing out where she was headed and what she seemed to want regarding her anxiety. During one of these sessions, Lulu had this extraordinary statement come out of her mouth. She said, "I want to leave my husband." She suddenly realized that anxiety was not her problem, though she certainly had it. Her problem was guilt. She said, "I remain in an abusive relationship based on my husband constantly guilt-tripping me and, through jealousy, treating me as an object that he can harass anytime he wants to." They both agreed to bring this up next week and give it their full attention. Lulu left the counselor's office feeling that the momentum was building for three or four weeks, but suddenly she had enough momentum to say what she needed to say.

The next week her counselor offered to help Lulu and her husband find a couple's counselor that could possibly help in working through their problems. As soon as Lulu's counselor mentioned this as a possibility, her heart sank and the momentum that had been building in her for that moment stopped. Her counselor, who was closely attuned to her at this point, realized that couple's counseling was not an option at that time. He then said, "OK, maybe I can help you work through the fallout from your experience with guilt and jealousy." The momentum was back on track, and that is how they spent the remaining sessions together.

In this case study, both a medical model and a more whole person model worked effectively. Both had a purpose and meaning in Lulu's life. The difference was the medical model had identified that she had an anxiety problem based on the diagnosis and treatment plan. However, regarding momentum, her experience with momentum was choppy at best. In her initial interview, momentum took hold but decreased during the diagnosis and treatment stages of counseling. It was only at the latter stages of practicing cognitive/behavioral techniques that she felt momentum start again.

However, by the time she left counseling, the momentum dropped off, except when she could use these skills in problems with her husband. It would be difficult to blame the medical model for not helping her with the relationship with her husband. She never really brought it up. However, she did not have enough momentum to address it—to get into a sticky area of her life.

Months later, she began feeling the anxiety returning. She found a counselor, but this time the counselor leaned more toward a holistic approach. From day one with the more holistic counselor, momentum began to grow. Their relationship was not based on fixing an anxiety problem. Their relationship was to help Lulu on her journey of self-discovery, wherever that would take her. As they began to develop a meaningful dialogue and her problems began to emerge, devising a plan was unnecessary. It developed itself, and Lulu's intuitive decision was to leave her husband. She had plenty of practice thinking about leaving, but she did not have the momentum to leave. Now the momentum was strong, and the possibility she chose was not to work on the relationship. In the end, she was empowered to solve her own problem, and that was partially based on gaining enough momentum in therapy to act on her own behalf.

One final note, the counselor could have encouraged her to seek couple's counseling based on that possibility being created. As someone who has worked with couples, if that was brought up near the beginning of counseling, I might have encouraged her to consider it without making that decision for her. However, this shows the power of momentum in the counseling process. The momentum she obtained during counseling was not only why she decided to leave her husband, but it was a part of her decision. Who is to say if she had focused on her husband early on whether things might have changed? In my experience, people tend to share information in therapy when they are ready to share it, and momentum seems to help in that process. That is unless a professional makes that decision for them while trying to help with their problems.

Medical Model and a Pattern of Momentum

Rapport Building

Rapport building may not be the initial process in a medical model, though in more progressive programs and clinics it is being used to gather information for an eventual diagnosis. Personally, it seems more associated with addiction, though I hope this continues to change regarding mental health.[2] In the previous case study, it was being used, and it does have the potential for creating momentum in a medical model. Motivational interviewing (MI), as used in the case study, is more of a humanistic, phenomenological technique based on the beliefs of Carl Rogers (Miller and Rollnick 2012). However, it is an effective beginning to create momentum with clients. It allows them to set the agenda while the interviewer listens and gives positive feedback to the client's story.

In contrast, many medical model programs have an initial interview that may not hold much weight for gaining momentum in therapy. Rather the information gathered is about making a diagnosis and treatment plan and logistical information for the business of mental health. This seems mandatory for many mental health programs but leaves little room for momentum. Since a medical model is a more natural scientific model and not a more phenomenological model, it is understandable why it does not hold as much importance in the opening moments of therapy.

Making a Diagnosis

As stated in other sections of this book, making a diagnosis is more involved with the mental health business through the *DSM-5* where professionals are looking for symptom probability to make the diagnosis as accurate as possible. Unfortunately, regarding momentum, making a diagnosis probably does not add any discernable momentum to the counseling process and sharing a diagnosis with a patient may cause a loss of momentum. Sharing a psychiatric label with patients runs the risk of them believing that it is who they are as a person, while making it harder for treatment in therapy.

Goal Setting

In a medical model, here would be a perfect place to set as one of the goals in therapy, the creation of momentum. I must say that in the forty years of practice, I have never seen a therapy goal based on creating momentum. However, during that time, in a more phenomenological model, momentum has been a primary consideration. For example, when counseling clients, if they need to miss a week, one of the first activities to accomplish is to reestablish momentum. If clients miss too many weeks, it may be wise to ask clients if they could help reestablish momentum, or is there something that is a roadblock to keeping the momentum going?

Intervention

It seems unfortunate that the chance for creating momentum needs to wait until counselors are faced with intervening into a client's problems with counseling techniques, homework assignments, or assignments of any kind. Having a certain level of momentum at the stage of intervention seems a mandatory practice in more holistic forms of therapy. I have seriously been baffled as to why medical model experts want to intervene with counseling skills based on their timetable rather than using momentum as a benchmark for when counseling skills could be effective. Practicing new skills and activities seems more effective with client momentum backing up practicing these skills than religiously following a treatment plan where the focus is on the counselor and not the client. Learning new techniques and skills is different than being in the right mood to use them.

Furthermore, I have observed many counseling skills and techniques being learned and practiced while using a medical model only to be forgotten when clients are on their own and return to their previous environment. The old system or environment may become bigger than the client in it. Without a certain level of momentum, it may be hard to continue practicing these skills when one's old world comes to reclaim them. The ability to have the momentum to fight through old patterns psychologically, socially, and neurologically may be the difference between working through a mental health problem for a new future versus having a temporary respite from experiencing problems based on the lack of consideration regarding momentum while practicing medical model therapy.

Termination

Without preserving a certain amount of momentum, termination may mean just that—ending therapy when one is still not able to be resilient enough to face the world. It seems difficult to gain momentum after going through therapy when the treatment plan was based on how to cope—as can be seen in some pharmaceutically based medical models. Coping is not growing and changing. For example, taking psychotropic drugs becomes the process of creating homeostasis or balance in clients/patients, which requires a minimal amount of momentum. It is no wonder the pharmaceutical companies have become so wealthy. Without momentum, many of the counseling skills and techniques may fall by the wayside and what is left are drugs. It takes virtually no momentum to take drugs if what you are using them for is to cope.

Phenomenological Model and a Pattern of Momentum

Develop Meaningful Dialogue

The earlier momentum is started in counseling, the better chance for it to successfully make a difference. As stated earlier in this chapter, momentum starts by building up a client's confidence in participating in the therapy process. For example, in the case study, Lulu met her counselor, and the unspoken rule was she could focus the session in any way she wanted to go. The counselor tried to empathize with Lulu's story while staying attuned to her as a person. Lulu's counselor had no intention of moving on until the therapeutic alliance was formed. In this manner, Lulu's counselor was practicing another theme connected to momentum. He was helping her get in touch with her competence as a person. She could see herself working together with her counselor to face her problems with anxiety and possibly other issues. By the end of establishing a meaningful dialogue, Lulu felt ready to proceed. Much like a football team where the coach pumps up the players to go out and fight for each other and victory, Lulu and her counselor gained enough momentum that would carry them from week to week in search of growth and change.

Let Problems Emerge

When Lulu went to the medical model clinic, there was little time for letting her problems emerge. They had identified the anxiety problem from the beginning and worked on a treatment plan to deal with it, and they successfully dealt with it. However, without any accumulated momentum, their success was only associated with the symptoms of Lulu's problems. It took a more phenomenological approach, based on looking at the whole person and gathering momentum around that person, for the problem facing Lulu to emerge. It is hard to say phenomenologically why the reason for Lulu's problem with her husband took so long to reveal itself. With momentum, one must realize something may take on a life of its own, and in this case, it was Lulu's husband. It could have been the freedom of letting Lulu free-associate while her counselor stayed attuned, practiced empathy, made intuitive decisions, or offered hope through selfless acts. Or, it could have been the momentum created in the ongoing experience that rushed her insightful and intuitive decision to leave her husband's conflict issues.

Develop an Action Plan

Here is where a medical model therapist and phenomenological counselor differ in a most important way. In a medical model, the therapist is acting as an expert and is called upon to develop an action plan that will relieve the symptoms that plague the patient. In a phenomenological model, the action plan is based on presenting possibilities to clients where they are empowered to decide for themselves, along with the help of the therapist. Making plans for one's future, even if it brings up personal fear, still is an experience where working through the fear creates even more momentum along with resilience.

When a client can own their plan, there is a sense of importance and responsibility to complete the plan. Having the momentum from meaningful dialogue through to acting out a client's personal plan creates more momentum for growth and change. With the support of a counselor, a client with momentum can weather adversity in the same way as an athletic team can come from behind to win a game. At a certain point, it becomes hard to determine whether you as a client have momentum or does the momentum have you? Are you riding on a wave of momentum that has affected your mood for growth and change (Yarrow, Brown, and Krakauer 2009)?

Practice

In the example of Lulu, there was no need to practice. She was going to leave her husband, and that was the road she took for her future. In other examples, after gaining momentum, it may become important to practice certain counseling techniques and skills until one feels comfortable with these skills and has gained momentum to use them. In practicing counseling and therapy, it seems more probable to practice these techniques and skills after gaining a level of momentum where the skills themselves add to the client's momentum.

There is another reason for practice, and it pertains to the myelin sheath that surrounds the axons on some nerve cells and forms an electrically insulating layer when constantly practicing certain procedures and experiences. Myelin is the fatty white substance that is essential for the proper functioning of the nervous system. It is an outgrowth of a type of glial cell that allows the embodied brain to act more efficiently (Siegel 2010). In athletes, practicing certain skills can increase their ability to be more efficient in said skills by becoming many times more efficient. Such practice can also add to any momentum taking place in athletics or in counseling. One other note regarding practice: A client does not have to limit practice to the outside world. Through mental imagery, a client can practice skills and techniques in their mind with equal results. Actual practice and mental practice of the same experience can create an equal amount of myelin growth (Bien 2006).

In a medical model, patients may be cognitively ready to practice counseling techniques and skills, but are they in the proper mood to sustain them? Having a history of gathering momentum as therapy progresses not only helps clients cognitively accept skills for their futures but also emotionally to perform these skills. You can use the same skills and the same procedures early in therapy when little or no momentum is present or use these techniques and skills at a level of momentum where even if the practice of these skills creates a certain level of fear, a client can use momentum to overcome these fears.

Growth and Change

Termination is a word used in medical model talk therapy that means symptoms have been reduced and the patient feels they have a level of skills to cope with life on their own. It is only if a person has a relapse, where the case is reopened, and another round of therapy begins. In a more phenomenological form of therapy, the goal is growth and change of a client as a whole person, and as a whole person, growth and change does not have to end when client and counselor stop seeing each other. A client can bring the momentum from counseling and apply it to other activities in life if the concept of momentum is thoroughly understood when clients leave counseling.

When I think about clients who have come back to therapy after a long stretch of being on their own, it seems to come down to two reasons overall. Either they come back because some overwhelming trauma has happened and they need the support of a counselor to listen to their problems, or they have run out of momentum and/or have lost it in some way. With the first example of overwhelming trauma, much like in a medical model, counseling may have to start from the beginning to work out where the client is at and what they want to do about it. However, more often, I find clients coming back based on running out of momentum, and with getting their momentum back, usually in one session, they jump back into the world to continue living their chosen life.

DISCUSSION

According to the research, it seems more obvious that the phenomenon of momentum is more visible and more noticeable in organized sports. I have often thought how magical the phenomenon of momentum is when out of nowhere a team comes to life to win a game. Maybe it is confidence. Maybe it is intrinsic motivation. Or, maybe it is momentum itself. To suddenly get a break in a game and realize, "We could win this!" and to be swept away by the momentum of the moment.

In counseling, the experience of momentum is subtle and not as visible. However, if one is looking for those nuances that make up a counseling session, it is present if you look for it. The flow of energy in the session seems to shift when something of importance happens. Alternatively, a client comes back the next session and appears different in their thoughts, emotions, or behavior. Or, suddenly there is a breakthrough insight where the client or the counselor puts everything that came before it into a different light.

Personally, I believe that momentum is created by our humanity when facing adversity. Such things as character, integrity, and courage kick in and will not let adversity win the day. Such confidence to face adversity and to gain momentum in one's life seems to come when we are in trouble in some way, and somewhere deep inside the choice is made to do something about it. I have seen this in clients when they believe in themselves and wanted to prove something to themselves and not necessarily to a talk therapist or anyone else.

NOTES

1. The concept and research on momentum primarily involves athletic events, so there are limited references in this chapter based on momentum, and counseling and momentum has not been researched in any depth. However, the phenomenon of momentum can be a large part of what happens in counseling either when momentum is gained or when it is lost. I have my personal list of what causes momentum, and they are guts (to face adversity), grit (to hang in there and not quit), risk (the willingness to risk), and zest (to think with compassion).

2. In treating individuals struggling with addiction, studies indicate that drug addiction treatment does not have to be voluntary to be effective. While clients may enter treatment involuntarily, motivational interviewing (MI) has shown to be effective in treating their addiction. By using MI treatment, we're able to embrace the spirit of MI, which is about "meeting the client where the client is" and can help nudge a client towards change by utilizing motivation enhancing techniques. *American Addiction Centers.*

Chapter Ten

Mindfulness and Phenomenology

There are similarities between mindfulness and phenomenology. Though many see mindfulness as a method, it is more than that. It can be a way of being in everyday life. Mindfulness is paying attention, on purpose, to our moment-to-moment unfolding experiences in the present in a nonjudgmental manner. It is becoming aware of emerging experiences. This facilitates a receptive stance towards our emerging thoughts, feelings, emotions, body sensations, and noticing what is present in our world (Nanda 2009).

If this seems familiar to what was stated in earlier chapters on attunement, insight, intuitive decision-making, momentum, and empathy—experientially, mindfulness and phenomenology are similar. Phenomenology aims to describe, understand, and interpret the meanings of experiences of human life. So mindfulness and phenomenology begin from a similar place. Both consider the art of observing experiences within ourselves both body and mind and within the world. For the talk therapist, it may be important to understand these phenomena when considering our connection to our clients.

NEUROSCIENCE, PHENOMENOLOGY, AND MINDFULNESS

For example, take the treatment of anxiety, which may be treated more effectively through bottom-up procedures rather than top-down procedures, namely the difference between the body responding to solving problems rather than the mind solving them.[1] Bottom-up procedures could begin phenomenologically by the therapist staying attuned to the client and waiting for intuitive decisions to emerge regarding the client's anxiety—both being bottom-up experiences. This can be followed by empathy and selfless acts presented by the therapist, with the goal being the formation of a therapeutic alliance. With an alliance formed, hope and humor can help in gathering momentum for the use of mindfulness techniques. At this point, the mindfulness technique of, for example, "focused breathing" could be introduced. With constant practice, this could reduce sympathetic nervous system arousal (Kabat-Zinn 2005). This also could reduce insular reactivity (Wheeler, Arnkoff, and Glass 2017) and improve emotional regulation. These processes do not take place in calculated decision-making but are more experiential, a bottom-up process for solving problems.

Many of the phenomenological themes from previous chapters reinforce the philosophy and practice of mindfulness techniques. With the increased popularity of mindfulness, it may be important to again point out the phenomenological method is experiential, not calculated. It is a method that allows phenomena to emerge. In many respects, so does mindfulness. For this reason, both mindfulness and phenomenology can be effective together in talk therapy (Felder and Robbins 2016). Figuring out a problem with top-down thinking may be no more effective than practicing mindfulness/phenomenological techniques that let problems emerge, so that client and counselor have an opportunity to solve them.

Mike was a person who loved hockey so much so that he gave up his law practice to help a university hockey team improve its results on the ice. However, if you would have asked what Mike was doing with the hockey players, most people would be curiously confused. His method of helping was phenomenological and, ultimately, based on mindfulness practices. Mike did not gather his players together and state that now they were going to practice breathing exercises based on mindfulness. He started out with phenomenology. He would sit down with players that were struggling and listen to them regarding their hockey performance, skill level, and the pressures they felt about winning. He stayed attuned to them and let decisions emerge regarding personal issues and performance. Some talked about their emotional struggle to feel confident on the ice, while others spoke about home life and the struggles affecting their ability.

Mike gave no answers during these individual meetings because his goal was to form an alliance. It was important for Mike that whatever skills his players practiced, they had a sense of ownership of them. So he took his time getting to know the players from many different angles. Empathy, selfless behavior, and creating hope were phenomena that one would not expect from a hockey coach. However, Mike was more than a coach. He was a person who used phenomenological counseling themes to get closer to his players.

Ultimately, he began teaching them mindfulness breathing exercises that were described as a method for improving performance with the team. However, phenomenology is a whole person experience that went beyond behavioral performance. The mindfulness breathing exercise was a way of forming a strong dialogue with his players. The one item Mike emphasized time and again was both mindfulness-oriented and phenomenological. The team had to practice this skill for one whole season until it became a part of them. He wanted the skill to gain momentum not only on the ice but also in their lives. University hockey still stayed competitive, but now it held another meaning for the players. It was a life skill that some of them used whether on the ice or not. Mike knew how to use phenomenology and mindfulness to help his hockey players not only be better players but also better people.

To make this story complete, let us map out how this combination of phenomenology and mindfulness was neurologically affecting the players. First, with the phenomenological introduction and the mindfulness follow-through, there probably was quite a bit of activity in the limbic area of the brain. The players most likely were learning to control the amygdala and its connection to the medial prefrontal cortex so the amygdala (the "crisis center") could not hijack the prefrontal cortex during a game. This combination could also help in emotional regulation so that the sympathetic nervous system had competition from the parasympathetic nervous system, and adrenaline would be used to make effective plays and not to overreact during a game. Such a combination probably affected their vagus nerve stimulation that runs almost the entire length of the body. Such a mindfulness technique could be used during warm-up where hockey players could sit on their hands while practicing deep breathing. This combination of phenomenological experiences combined with mindfulness skills, all coming more from the gut rather than the head, was a strategy that worked for Mike.

The question that one could ask is, "How does all this fit into talk therapy?" First, the phenomenological themes discussed in this example are not counseling skills but human experiences. Practicing intuitive decision-making, empathy, or insight is not the ownership of counseling or psychology. They are phenomena that come out of experience regardless of the circumstances taking place in the world. Regarding mindfulness, it also is not limited to counseling or psychology skills, though many mindfulness skills are practiced in these areas. Mindfulness also comes from an experiential frame of mind that is practiced by such religions as Buddhism but also in those observers of experience that want to understand phenomena without any judgments or hypotheses.

However, one thing seems obvious. Mindfulness skills and phenomenological experiences come more from bottom-up problem-solving rather than top-down attempts to solve problems. It may be that some of the phenomenological experiences being demonstrated in this book can be used under the label of mindfulness skills. When practicing intuitive decision-making, or experiencing momentum in counseling, or bracketing emotions through empathy, there can be a similar experience as practicing breathing exercises or meditation. Though these phenomenological experiences may seem more active than some mindfulness skills, they seem to be coming from the same place—the embodied brain—and they seem to bring someone to personal integration (Siegel 2016).[2] There is little reason to figure out in mindfulness or phenomenology what is happening. It is a matter of letting whatever is happening emerge.

PHENOMENOLOGICAL EXPERIENCES USED AS MINDFULNESS

In the following sections, let us look at how some of the phenomenological experiences described in this book can be used as mindfulness. Neurologically and phenomenologically, these themes need clarification within a more phenomenological model of talk therapy. Since the therapeutic alliance has been proven to be one of the most important experiences in talk therapy, and since many of the experiences needed to obtain that alliance are more phenomenological than natural scientific, let us cast these experiences into the realm of mindfulness. For example, let us see intuitive decision-making as a form of mindfulness or empathy and momentum as mindfulness phenomena. Even though many of the themes in this book are not usually identified as mindfulness, let us now identify them that way. The philosophical underpinning of both is not that different. There are many similarities between Buddhism and mindfulness on one side and phenomenology and existentialism on the other (Colaizzi 1978).

Phenomenology or Mindfulness?

Intuition

Intuition as a mindfulness technique makes sense from a phenomenological and neurological perspective. Neurologically, the ventromedial prefrontal cortex can elicit the emotional responses that people deem as gut feelings or hunches (Bechara, Damasio, Damasio, and Lee 1999). Combine this with the locus coeruleus, a minute nucleus located in the pons in the middle brain, and this combination is said to generate one's gut feelings. The reason is that the pons area supplies noradrenaline to the forebrain, which influences emotion, motivation, memory, learning, and decision-making, and because of this, it also plays a role in the experience of intuition (Demasio 2005).

In mindfulness, you have a similar neurological experience. However, more importantly, it is how the brain is experiencing a person's experiences that make the difference. There are two networks to consider in mindfulness. (These are more phenomenologically described than neurologically, but both are helpful to understand mindfulness.) The first is what is called the "narrative network" (Rock 2009).[3] This is the network of thinking when there really is little to think about. In counseling and therapy, this network sometimes can get clients into trouble based on thinking about anything and everything, such as ruminating about anxiety, relatives, and anything else with a narrative story that could be running through one's mind. The opposite may also be true. Such thinking can be creative, help organize problems, and help us understand one's personal narrative of the world. When you experience the world using this narrative network, you take in information from the outside world, process it through a filter of what everything means, and add your interpretations (Rock 2009). This neural network makes up most of our thinking.

However, there is a whole other way a person is experiencing his or her experiences. The second network is called the "direct experience network" and includes the insula, a region that relates to perceiving bodily sensations. The anterior cingulate cortex is also activated, which is a region of the brain central to switching your attention. When this direct experience network is activated, you are not thinking intently about the past or future, other people, or yourself, or considering much at all. Rather, you are experiencing information coming into your senses in real time (Singleton et al. 2014). What some phenomenologists would call a disciplined naïveté (Spinelli 2005). Through this direct experience network, mindfulness can help distill mental rumination, help weigh options, tune into your intuition, and, ultimately, make decisions that you can stand behind. By using mindfulness, intuitive decision-making becomes more of continued practice than an isolated event.

As a rule, the medical model relies on calculated decisions, and in many respects, experienced mental health professionals can be quite accurate at making these decisions. However, in the world of phenomenology, intuitive decision-making fits more with a non-hypothesis model where a decision is made from the bottom-up and intuitively. In counseling and therapy, it is not difficult to make intuitive decisions. It is a matter of letting the embodied brain guide you to the correct answer. Mindfulness also is not difficult. The hard part is remembering to do it. It takes practice (Rock 2009). Sometimes in a medical model, fulfilling treatment plans, or initiating certain counseling skills may not allow a counselor time to listen for those intuitive and mindful moments. Those moments in mindfulness and phenomenology, when focusing intently on what is being said by clients, activates the direct experience network where counselors intensely focus on what is in front of them.

Annmarie made a point that before sitting down with a client, she would do five minutes of breathing exercises. She would comment that, "It was my way of clearing my head of assumptions, chatter, and any outside thoughts that would implicate a breakdown in my intuitive decision-making." She rarely had an agenda when speaking with her clients. She wanted to stay attuned to what was going on in front of her. This was different than some of her colleagues who seemed to have a plan of action ready when meeting with their clients. At times, other colleagues would say she was ill-prepared, yet her waiting list of clients was longer than anyone else. Annmarie practiced mindfulness skills at home but practiced different mindfulness in counseling. She knew when to be mindful of others, and they appreciated it.

Attunement

Mirror neurons are firings from the client's brain to the counselor's brain, helping both comprehend and bridge the gap between what is going on from one mind to the other. In the brain, the pathway that makes all this happen starts with the insula portion of the brain, which is responsible for self-awareness and subjective emotions (Craig 2009). At this point, the phenomenon called the "emotional moment" allows the body and mind of both client and counselor to be subjectively aware of their present moments in counseling (Craig 2009). These firings also become connected to what is happening in the client's and counselor's bodies that will go through the emotional processing center of the limbic system, which will send signals to the prefrontal cortex for an emotional act to take place (Berlucchi and Aglioti 1997). In therapy, this neurological process ends up with the counselor knowing what the client is feeling and the client having a similar reaction to the feelings of the counselor (Bozarth 2009).

This previously stated description of attunement can be applied in phenomenological experiences but also in mindfulness experiences as well. In mindfulness, when staying attuned to a certain object, person, or thought for any length of time, a mindfulness "emotional moment" can also take place. There is an attunement where a person is connected differently through this unique experience. People who meditate are familiar with this experience, which is when a calming effect comes over them and much of the world'ss chaos and rigidity leaves their thoughts and emotions.

Phenomenologically, in counseling, a similar connection happens with counselors where they become attuned to where the client is at—not ahead of the client or behind the client, but presently with the client. It can be argued that such an experience can be described as mindfulness where you are not attuned to an object or thing but to another human being and where you are experiencing directly what is presently happening. Such a mindfulness focus can sometimes resonate immediately with the client. It is a connection that bonds client and counselor together and can be a part of what more progressive neuroscientists call integration (Siegel 2016).

Empathy

Empathy becomes a combination of integration between the supramarginal gyrus, hippocampus, and amygdala but also the second brain of the client, which is called the gut. Empathy depends on the gut to send signals to the cerebral cortex to not only gather objective information but also subjective information, especially emotional information. The brain in your head isn't your only brain. There's a "second brain" in your intestines that contains a hundred million neurons. Gut bacteria are responsible for making over thirty neurotransmitters including serotonin (Carpenter 2012). What makes empathy so powerful in the practice of counseling is its ability to integrate the supramarginal gyrus, cerebral cortex, mirror neurons, amygdala, hippocampus, and the gut when listening and responding to clients.

This previous description of empathy from a neurological perspective shows the power of the integration between mind and body when empathizing with others. Much like attunement, empathy seems to favor a more gut-based activity rather than a logic-based practice. In bracketing one's thoughts and feelings and absorbing the thoughts and feelings of another, it seems to have strong implications for letting go of assumptions, judgments, analysis, and so forth and focusing directly on the present. Thus it turns out that empathy may be one of the strongest mindfulness techniques used in counseling or therapy. This may be why it becomes difficult for those who are "trying to empathize." Much as in mindfulness training, it is the power of letting go and having the present emerge where meaning is found.

The client, Luke, brought up so many issues that it seemed impossible to know what was going on with this client. He spoke nonstop for forty-five minutes with countless scenarios being put out for the counselor to absorb. At the end of all this, the counselor stated, "Being that lonely in all these situations must be a sad life." Luke began to cry and admitted it was what the client was trying to convey. Here is an accurate example of empathy being used as mindfulness. Instead of focusing on the forty-five minutes of drama vented by the client, the counselor focused on one traumatic theme—the loneliness in each story—not wavering and not trying to follow anything else. This is similar to more typical mindfulness exercises where one focuses on one thing and, when distracted, constantly brings the focus back to that one thing. This becomes difficult to accomplish in empathy and in other mindfulness when distracted by outside issues. Luke said in numerous ways, "I am lonely." So the counselor responded through empathy to this call for help. Instead of trying to figure out what each story was all about, the counselor allowed the theme of loneliness to emerge.

Selflessness

Some of the principles of phenomenology and mindfulness come together in selfless acts. In mindfulness, the idea is to keep one's attention for extended periods of time outside of one's self. Usually, this attention can be on an object, or one's breath, or our usual perception of ourselves. To get outside ourselves beyond what we accept as our core identity. For example, in therapy, it is not the counselor, Peter, focusing on the client's anxiety, but Peter perceiving himself outside of himself when viewing the client's anxiety.

I must share with you the first time this phenomenon of selflessness took hold of me. A Kenyan poet would, on occasion, share her poetry with me. Once, she read a poem about this princess who was in the mirror in front of her. She described the beauty of her skin, the shape of her body, and many other explicit details. The poem was remarkable. It was genuinely fantastic, but for one Western world perception made by me. I told her that the poem was beautiful but was it not a bit egotistical? From my Western world perspective, I made this conclusion. If she wrote the poem about the princess in the mirror, then the princess in the mirror must be her. She laughed and said the princess in the mirror had nothing to do with her. She was not talking about herself but the image of the person in the mirror. She had selflessly detached her identity from what she saw in front of her. This is a practice that people practicing mindfulness do all the time. It also describes a disciplined naïveté for observing phenomena in the everyday world. Selfless acts in life, or selfless acts in therapy, have an intensity of seeing objects, emotions, and other behaviors for themselves and not from what we have learned to see through our experiences. My only defense in this example was that I still was clinging to my empirical perception of the world and did not see the poem for itself.

How many times have I observed successful therapists and counselors make the same mistake? From a more empirical perspective, for example, if you see the guidelines presented from the *DSM-5* regarding an anxious person, then the focus is on one's self and the knowledge you have acquired from personal experience and *DSM* guidelines. However, from a phenomenological perspective and, I might add, from a mindfulness perspective, the anxious client takes on a perception uniquely their own. By the counselor getting outside of his or her self, it does not become what the counselor sees for one's self but for what is there, in the present world, in front of the counselor demonstrating the client's anxiety in a unique way. From such selfless acts, counselors not only encourage but set the stage for intuitive acts, attunement, and empathy to take place.

A mindful perception of the world becomes very similar to a phenomenological worldview when one goes beyond one's self. Paradoxically, by doing this, one becomes more attuned with the world and, ultimately, the world reveals itself when practicing the art of being selfless and other-directed. It becomes not what the therapist knows about the client but what is perceived about the client in his or her world. For example, if clients say the buildings are falling, then a counselor should perceive the buildings falling and stay focused on such perceptions to understand the experiential world of the client, rather than concluding that such a client is simply paranoid. From our world, the client may be paranoid, but from the client's world, the buildings are falling down.

Insight

Insight links the past, present, and future. Insight means integrating cortical representation of autobiographical memory stores and limbic firing that gives emotional texture to the emerging themes of our present awareness, life story, and image of the future (Siegel 2010). In other words, insight puts together a collection of memories along with spurts of emotion to create emotional meaning to what the client is experiencing regarding the present, past life stories, and images of the future. From a phenomenological perspective, insight helps clients understand how events in their past are currently influencing their current thoughts, emotions, and behaviors along with an understanding of how these insights can affect future events. Insights not only help with awareness, but they also help with meaning during a counseling session.

In understanding mindfulness, it would be hard to make the argument that insight is a part of mindfulness. Mindfulness is about being in the present and attuned to something other than one's historical self. Insight is a culmination of past, present, and future where new meaning is found through the integration of all three experiences in time. However, mindfulness separates mindless chatter and creates a disciplined focal point that can produce a calming effect throughout the integrated mind (Bien 2006). In other words, mindfulness can set the stage for insight to take place. Intuition, attunement, empathy, and selfless acts as mindfulness set the stage for the past, present, and future to come together in some "*aha!* moment."

It may be surprising to some people how much useless chatter takes place in one's mind during the day. Add this to the rumination that goes on with such things as mood disorders or anxiety disorders, and it makes sense that insightful moments do not happen with any amount of frequency. However, mindfulness may be of value by clearing the way for valuable insights to emerge. If clients can get by all the useless chatter that adds to their problems, then a pathway is made for these insights. Mindfulness can clear that pathway.

George had difficulty remembering the past and how he ended up reluctantly admitting that he hated himself. All he really knew was that while in his family of origin, he felt like a second-class citizen. This haunted him into his late twenties until he decided to seek counseling. His counselor took the first number of sessions trying to follow an overabundance of information from his past but with little success. Finally, George's counselor decided to collaborate with him on trying mindfulness training, and George agreed. After practicing mindfulness for a month, George's mind was not as full of useless chatter, and the thoughts that were left had clarity and purpose.

Finally, George had a "spontaneous moment" where he realized members of his family rejected him for his mixed-race background. George's parents never gave that impression after he was adopted, but his brothers and sisters subtly made that point to him as he was growing up. Before practicing mindfulness, those thoughts about his siblings came to his mind more than once, but there was so much useless chatter in his mind that having such thoughts stand out seemed an impossibility. It was only after mindfulness that George came to that insight.

Momentum

In this example, George suffered from self-hatred, which led him to counseling. Sometimes through anxiety, depression, or trauma, a deeper sense of self is uncovered. If George had any of these symptoms, they were attributed to this underlying identity crisis of self-hatred. However, even with his counselor practicing empathy, attunement, and the selfless act of positive regard, the amount of mindless chatter that George had to experience while trying to solve this problem made it difficult for any insight to emerge. The agreed upon mindfulness exercises changed that problem. Through repetition of mindfulness, George gained momentum and confidence until much of the chatter in his mind had disappeared. He began to clear his mind of useless chatter. Now insight and other revelations were in a better position to emerge. Such an example shows the power of mindfulness, not necessarily to solve a problem, but to clear the air around a problem so it can emerge as a matter of insight.

However, mindfulness and looking at the world from a phenomenological perspective have one important aspect in common. Both need a certain level of practice. As stated earlier, we mostly live in a narrative network of experience, and George, in the former example, was a victim of this narrative way of thinking. So changing to a more experiential, in the present, network of experience may only have a chance of working if George keeps practicing mindfulness. Awareness is not enough with mindfulness. It takes practice until it seems more commonplace within someone's world.

From a neurological perspective, practice helps rewire one's neuropathways, and with extended practice, it helps in the development of a more efficient set of mindfulness skills. Neurologically, it creates growth and modulation of synaptic connections among neurons creating different neurological connections—in other words, it rewires negative neuropathways to positive neuropathways, especially in the anterior cingulate (Bush, Luu, and Posner 2000). Secondly, it helps to lay down a myelin sheath around neural transmitters, increasing action potential of ions to move much faster—neuropathways become faster and more productive (Patoine 2016).

Finally, practice creates momentum, and momentum creates confidence, perceived competence, and intrinsic motivation (Kabat-Zinn 2005). Keeping the momentum after counseling has ended becomes a high priority for the more phenomenological counselors. This might be why clients working with more holistic counselors who practice mindfulness skills keep their momentum phenomenologically as whole people, but also have gained momentum in the use of mindfulness. Along with diet and exercise, mindfulness skills may be a reason for keeping one's momentum going in continued growth and change after counseling.

DISCUSSION

There are differences between phenomenology, existentialism, mindfulness philosophy, humanistic psychology, and other whole person-oriented schools of thought that benefit from a more human science in the field of mental health. There are more natural scientific schools of thought, such as behaviorism, some cognitive schools, and most of psychiatry. All have made an impact on the mental health profession. In some respects, mindfulness has helped more humanistic schools of thought, especially with its popularity.

It was important in this chapter to point out that not all mindfulness skills come specifically from some form of actual skills presented on their own, such as breathing exercises, meditation, EMDR, or any other mindfulness activity. However, let us not forget that within procedures of phenomenology are embedded mindfulness-oriented skills that sometimes go unrecognized as mindful. Intuitive decision-making has connections to mindfulness in it is bottom-up problem-solving. Attunement uses the practice needed in using a more experiential neurological network as does mindfulness in staying attuned to clients. In empathy, one needs to bracket both thoughts and behavior, therefore demonstrating a similar practice in mindfulness of leaving your identity behind when perceiving an object, thought, or person. Both selfless acts and mindfulness also leave the self behind when connecting to an outside focus. Moreover, even though insight probably lies in the more narrative network rather than the experiential network of perceiving the world, it holds a certain level of effectiveness when mindfulness clears out many of the thoughts and chatter that disrupt a person from having insights. In the field of phenomenological talk therapy, I believe it is important to credit mindfulness as one of many phenomenological techniques that help clients grow and change. My personal experience is in using mindfulness as a part of a phenomenological approach to talk therapy.

NOTES

1. Much of what is considered bottom-up thinking refers to intuition and insights being initiated more from one's gut feelings than from a more logical rational origination such as the mind. In this book, many of the themes found in each chapter come from bottom-up thinking. A more natural scientific way of thinking can be called top-down thinking based on making a

hypothesis and then trying to prove its validity. Ladd, Peter D. and AnnMarie Churchill. 2012. *Person-Centered Diagnosis and Treatment in Mental Health: A Model for Empowering Clients*. London, UK: Jessica Kingsley Publishing, 1-25.

2. Personal integration was discussed in Chapter 2. The basic understanding of this phenomenon is stated by Daniel Siegel; the mind is an emergent, self-organizing, embodied, and relational process that regulates the flow of energy and information. Mind emerges out of energy and information that flows through our interpersonal connections, our brain, and whole body (embodied brain), where this energy and information self-organizes all at once and in all directions. What emerges from this spontaneous interaction, we call the "mind." All these parts create a system where experience can emerge. However, the parts of the mind are not the cause of experiences emerging. It is the interplay within this system where experiences can emerge on their own. Siegel, Daniel. 2016. *Mind: A Journey to the Heart of Being Human*. New York, NY: W.W. Norton & Company.

3. The terms narrative network and direct experience network are not neurological terms. They refer to the two types of experiences we have when our brain is active. The narrative network is what drives us most of the time. We are constantly having thoughts and feelings going through our minds about the past, present, and future and how we relate to these experiences in everyday life. The experiential network refers more to stopping the narrative network by focusing on something outside of our usual narrative, such as found in mindfulness.

Chapter Eleven

Hope

Talk Therapy's Ultimate Goal

NEUROSCIENCE AND HOPE

The latest research, based on studies of placebos given to subjects in mental health research, reveals that hope can affect the brain to alleviate a range of serious afflictions, including pain, Parkinson's disease, and depression (Alexander 2017). One of the interesting issues for phenomenological talk therapists is how a procedure used more for medical research, the "placebo effect," can demonstrate the power of hope when introduced into counseling or therapy. For example, patients who took placebos in numerous studies believed their mental health would improve when they thought they were taking some form of psychotropic medication, and remarkably, they did improve (Carlson 2015). In talk therapy, the power of meaningful beliefs may hold possibilities regarding the importance of creating hope for clients in the therapy process.

Here is research from Zubieta and Stohler that make this point. Hope boosts our own capacity to suppress pain by employing the brain's own "anti-pain" mechanisms—the endogenous opioids, or endorphins, causing observable changes in the brain. Endorphins—the brain's own (endogenous) morphine—are released during stress or during sustained pain to regulate those experiences (Zubieta and Stohler 2009). These results indicate that when we believe in something meaningful, the connection between mind and body begin to work together. From a neurological perspective, hope uses the same chemical pathways in the brain as chemically active analgesics to reduce pain, improve health, and a feeling of well-being (Benedetti, Carlino, and Pollo 2011).

Furthermore, hope seems more than a vague abstraction. It appears to have a practical purpose in talk therapy. From a whole person perspective, hope taps into a client's natural ability to heal. However, our pursuit of creating hope in clients is quite different than using a placebo in medical model research. The placebo has been used to point out the effectiveness of such things as the effects of drugs on subjects by using a control group where, for example, placebos are given out but without full disclosure to the subjects. Such natural scientific procedures may not be conducive to the spirit behind a more phenomenological model.

From the beginning, it may be important to fully describe how hope works in the healing process during therapy. The question may come down to, "How can a client with a negative outlook on life find an authentic sense of hope even before resolving their issues?" This may lead to the therapist creating a meaningful dialogue when a client enters with a negative outlook toward therapy. It may make sense to describe the experience of hope from a more neurophenomenological viewpoint, where the experience of hope is backed up by neuroscience. However, beyond neuroscience is the connection between therapist and client where their meaningful dialogue together from moment to moment, allow trust, hope, and belief to emerge, and, in so doing, we are working with an innate human ability to heal (Carlson 2015).

Elizabeth came to counseling saying that she really did not have a problem but wanted to discuss a situation that had surfaced in her life. She described being asked by her father if she could help take care of her mother who was seriously ill. Her relationship with her father was always considered warm and affectionate, yet with her mother, a long history of abuse lingered in the background. She had not been close to her mother for a long time and had not even visited her over the years based on what Elizabeth considered an abusive childhood. Now that her parents were in their eighties, much had happened over the years, yet Elizabeth never forgot how her mother physically and emotionally abused her. The abuse became so bad that when she was in her teens she struck out on her own. The passing years were kind to her based primarily on her intelligence and motivation. She held many important jobs, graduated from an Ivy League institution, and was at a point where all she needed to do was finish a dissertation and she would earn a PhD.

Her therapist, Sidney, asked, what exactly did she want out of the therapy process. Elizabeth said that she found it difficult caring for her mother based on her early childhood and that resentment and anger kept building up inside of her now that their roles were reversed. She admitted that her childhood trauma was not worked through in any complete fashion, but the hurt was all brought back now that she was caring for her mother. Elizabeth felt hopeless and stuck in a situation that made her start to question herself and her success. She felt like a victim of abuse and started questioning the success that she had accomplished after leaving her parent's home.

Numerous sessions were spent discussing her victimization and the hurt she felt that was connected to the past. To Elizabeth, the situation felt hopeless no matter how much she talked about it. Sidney decided to use his form of phenomenological therapy by making a comparison between a lover, a lumberjack, and a botanist. He said that when the lover looks at a big oak tree, she sees a place to carve a heart in it as a witness of love for her boyfriend. The lumberjack looks at the same tree and sees how many board feet could come out of the tree. The botanist looks at the same tree and sees the formation of the leaves and how they compare to other trees. These people are looking at the same tree but seeing it differently (Ladd 2016).

Sidney said to Elizabeth, "When you tell your story of victimization, I picture a different story. For me, it is a story of triumph and survival. Beyond the abuse, you were able to pull yourself together and make something of your life. It seems to me you are in a position of helping your mother, not as a victim of her abuse but as a survivor of it. Furthermore, looking at it as a survivor also affects changes both experientially and neurologically. By looking at the experience of taking care of your mother as a proud survivor, you begin to neurologically start to rewire your brain towards being hopeful and not hopeless. From where I am sitting, your story only makes sense to me from the point of view of hope. Who knows what will come out of the experience with your mother if you consider changing your point of view. Maybe even reconciliation."

Elizabeth eventually decided to make a change. Not based on Sidney telling her to change her viewpoint but based on Sidney's view giving her a sense of hope. She spent the next few months taking care of her mother until her death. She commented to others about how lucky she was to have the chance to reconcile with her before she passed away. She now, when thinking of her mother, was not peering into the past but thinking about the new foundation she had for the future. When looking at her past, she felt hopeful that there were lessons in it, and not all of them placed her in the role as victim. Elizabeth had rewritten the past with a new theme centered on hope. She saw her mother still as abusive but in a more compassionate way.

One may look at this example and say there were no counseling techniques used and using metaphors may be a bit off target regarding Elizabeth's problems. From a phenomenological perspective, when finding a way to help clients heal, not all treatment has to be formulated around any medical model established technique or predetermined goal. A keen observer of counseling techniques may say that Sidney was using metaphors as a counseling technique and narrative therapy to reframe Elizabeth's story. However, these were not preplanned, calculated decisions based on a treatment plan but intuitive decisions that spoke to Elizabeth as a whole person and not to her symptoms.

This also is a prime example of therapist as educator. It is hard for clients to make accurate decisions regarding their future without relevant information. Sidney set the stage for Elizabeth to decide what she wanted to do regarding her mother. He set the stage by giving her an alternative based on hope. As we will see later in this chapter, hope is a transfer of energy and purpose from one experience to another more favorable one.

From a neurological perspective, Sidney's attunement and insight also allowed changes to Elizabeth's brain chemistry. The results show that "placebos" decrease activity in certain areas of the brain—namely the thalamus, insula, and anterior cingulate cortex (Wager 2004). These regions become active during pain and the anticipation of pain and are also influenced by analgesic medications—thus providing further evidence that pharmacologically active drugs and placebo treatment-induced positive expectations activate the same pain-modulation networks (Wager et al. 2004). Obviously, this research is not directly connected to the phenomenon of hope; however, anticipatory expectations are the common ground between hope and the placebo effect. Both anticipate a positive change in one's future: placebos through some designated drug, and hope through some new and different vision of the past, present, or future. Elizabeth decided to "buy in" to Sidney's future view of the relationship between mother and daughter.

PHENOMENOLOGY AND HOPE

In trying to understand phenomenological research, it may be important to show the difference between this form of research and natural scientific research. In natural scientific research, the researcher is looking to discover facts or a reasonable statistical significance, such as whether a certain drug can alleviate pain. Natural scientific research also may be interested in looking to discover probability in certain phenomena, such as in the *DSM-5* research on disorders surrounding pain. Phenomenological research is more holistic in that it is looking more for possibilities that can relate to the whole person. For example, through hope, it is possible to relieve pain in someone like Elizabeth who is trying to face a problem with her mother (Bullington 2009).[1] The goal of certain phenomenological research is invested in quality research based on nuances emerging during the dialogue between client and counselor and not captured through natural science.

For example, in the above story about Sidney using the tree metaphor or telling his version of Elizabeth's story during therapy, it is not easily quantifiable, and the efficacy through natural science of both examples does not match their effectiveness (Larsen, Edey, and Lemay 2007) . However, they are effective in creating the possibility for hope growing in Elizabeth. Hope is a phenomenon that goes beyond an understanding through quantifiable research. Hope is a part of what makes us human and is uniquely ours and cannot be empirically reduced to fit in with characteristics of anyone else. However, if we find true meaning in our experience with hope, we can change our beliefs and subsequently change our brains. Hope offers the possibility of changing the neuropathways in our brains, where our experience of hope enters into a reciprocal relationship with our brain's neuropathways, ultimately expressing hope where one reinforces the other. This reciprocal relationship creates a sense of intentionality, and it helps us stay directed toward a meaningful future.

Another issue to discuss might be the importance of separating hope from expectations. For example, unreasonable expectations can quash thoughts of hope when expected outcomes do not come true. Hope is not necessarily a goal. It is more in line with an aspiration. It reflects a desire, a yearning, an eagerness, and a longing (Webster's Dictionary 2017). Hope points you in a direction away from hopelessness, away from misery, sorrow, anguish, and desperation (Webster's Dictionary 2017). In the case of Elizabeth, Sidney did not set medical model-oriented goals for her or create any expectations. He simply stated how he perceived the situation with her mother. One cannot assume that Sidney's explanation of brain chemistry regarding hope or his metaphor regarding the tree or his version of Elizabeth's story was the difference in Elizabeth helping her mother. Such phenomena are difficult to quantify without losing the nuances that make them unique. However, possibly all of them may have been involved. In Elizabeth's case, creating hope through different possibilities was present in the information shared in therapy and this, along with other possibilities, led to her insightful decision.

Hope may be difficult to quantify, but it has no problem being practical. In as simple terms as possible, hope is taking something that is not working and transferring one's energy into something that shows promise to work. Hope is not a high-level abstraction pertaining to some mystical reality, for example, "I hope within my dreams that things will change." From a phenomenological perspective, hope holds the intentionality for change (May 1969).[2] In other words, we are always conscious of something out in the world , but if you do not know what that is, then you will not be able to act on it. In the case study, Sidney made aware to Elizabeth a new story, a new perception of her mother, so if Elizabeth wanted, she could act on it.

Here is where phenomenology needs clarification. In phenomenology, one does not have to be deliberate about your intent as you normally are, for example, in coming up with a medical model treatment plan. Intentionality understood within phenomenology is already there for you. You cannot avoid it (Knut 2009). Sidney, in the case study, did not intend to have Elizabeth "buy in" to his example of the story about her mother. He wanted to put it out there so that she could not avoid it—to decide whether she would give it purpose and meaning in her life, as a distinct possibility. Phenomenological counselors sometimes show clients a different perception of reality, in this case, the reality of hope, so they can decide whether to make something of meaning for themselves. Intentionality describes the continual correlation between the subject and the object, which, in this case, is Elizabeth and how she plans to view her mother.

Changing the intentionality in therapy to what the therapist wants the client to accomplish may indirectly take hope out of the experience and replace it with control (Chamodraka, Fitzpatrick, and Janzen 2017). In some cases, trying to control the outcome of therapy can be counterintuitive—the more control, the less positive can be the results. On the other hand, through intentionality of the client, hope can create a picture of the future where the possibility for healing exists. Our hopes for the future do not have to be organized in our minds through checklists, linear steps, specific goals, or treatment plans. Hope needs the breathing room of something for the future that is important to us. As therapists, we cannot create hope in clients by walking them through standardized steps to achieve what they are looking to get out of therapy.

Even counseling techniques need to be offered as possibilities and not as interventions or mandates to follow. In my experience, I have not run across many successful standardized formulas for successful therapy without considering the hopes and dreams of the client. Clients and therapist's hopes and dreams may need to be intermingled with a new creative experience where both client and therapist believe the experience is meaningful. Hope for the future is not necessarily based on controlling the future. Sometimes it is important to trust the process of therapy when two like-minded people have hope for an agreed upon and acceptable future.

Hope is about the future having an impact on the present while considering what has happened in the past. Hope connects the past, present, and future in a new creative way. In counseling, I have seen clients find hope in the future and, during the moment of experiencing it, having them change with a new acceptance, a different view of the present and past. In this regard, I believe that hope is transformative, possibly even life-changing. Such moments in therapy are impossible to measure empirically.

PHENOMENOLOGICAL PATTERN OF HOPELESSNESS

For some people, hopelessness is based on being unable to envision a future. This is relevant in those people who consider suicidal behavior. In the following section, before looking at the phenomenological pattern of hope, it may be important to compare hope with hopelessness. The following case study will help as a guide.

Jim had no clear perception of his future after he, yet again, experienced another bout of depression. This was the fourth experience with it in his forty-eight years on the planet. He had grown accustomed to the feelings that slowly came over him, usually after months of stressful experiences. He believed that depression caused him shame, especially with his family and his inability to go to work and make a living. However, Jim showed no real interest in many things. Those experiences that used to bring him joy were gone: playing with his children, discussions with his wife, walking the dog. These daily rituals seemed obliterated by this cloudy and debilitating view of his future. Irrationally, he saw no real future; he would add up all the experiences in life that he should feel grateful for, yet he felt more shame than gratefulness.

It seemed that each time he went through a bout of depression, the future became more uncertain and more vague and unrecognizable. It was as though he was caught in a bubble where beyond the bubble was some semblance of a life, but the bubble kept him from experiencing it. This is how Jim saw the world: caught in his present misery, depressed and feeling alone, even though his family was present, ready, and willing to help him. However, Jim did not want their help. He believed that he had let them down and it was time to help himself, even though he had little understanding of what he could do.

Finally, he went to his family doctor, who put him on an SSRI. In the first few weeks, he felt even more helpless because he was anticipating some radical change in his condition, a change that did not come. After a few weeks, he did feel some relief. However, his ego about being a depressed person simply lowered his symptoms but did not take away his sense of helplessness. He would say to himself, "Why haven't the drugs taken care of this? What else is wrong with me that I feel like there is nothing I can do to get out of these feelings?"

Feeling helpless was the tone of any conversation Jim held with others. "What is wrong with me? Why can I not snap out of this on my own?" In previous bouts with depression, he made similar claims and felt worthless and became overly sensitive to anyone bringing up the topic of his depression. On the one hand, Jim felt helpless, but he did not want to talk about accepting any help. He began to believe his future would be filled with similar experiences, and he could not see himself in this helpless position once again.

With each bout of depression, he viewed his possibilities for the future shrinking, even though he refused to get help from a counselor or therapist. He had become complacent in his bubble. He wanted to stay there until the depression lifted, as he slowly found himself slipping away from an ability to work, an ability to communicate, and an ability to feel anything but emotional pain. Moreover, the pain seemed like the only experience that was significantly changing. It was obliterating his future. It was making any attempts at pulling out of the depression a distant waning possibility.

There came a point where he had retreated from the caring people in his life. However, he did not care anymore. Life had lost its meaning. It seemed like an endless experience of emotional pain. He had gotten to the point where life felt meaningless, and the pain was all that he could bear. He began to lose hope, and his hopelessness led him to an attempt at suicide through overdosing on pills. Fortunately, his wife did not give up on him and immediately rushed him to the hospital where he was treated for his suicide attempt. After this, Jim reluctantly agreed to see a mental health therapist about his present condition.

A Pattern of Hopelessness

No Clear View of the Future

For those who find themselves feeling hopeless, it is difficult to believe they have a clear view of the future where they are prepared for possible upcoming traumatic events. It seems more likely that hopelessness starts with a vague perception of future experiences and events. When feeling hopeless, a person is more inclined to react rather than act. We see this with Jim in the case study. He had no clear view of the future where he could counteract depressed feelings. Hopelessness is not a phenomenon that has you reaching out for an understanding of a future. A person becomes wrapped up in vague and confusing experiences in the present, let alone seeing clearly what is important as preparation for future events. There is little time and place to take a stand on future events when it seems difficult to take a stand on the present.

Feeling of Helplessness

It becomes a helpless feeling to find yourself drifting into a future without experiencing an inner sense of control over that future.[3] Not in the sense that someone needs to have complete control over the future, but a feeling of control over one's self when entering an unpredictable future. As many existentialist writers have stated, we are thrown into our experiences, but it is up to us to choose how we will deal with them (Frankl 2014; Heidegger 1996). In cases of depression, as stated in the above example, many clients cannot clearly visualize a future, which may trigger a sense of helplessness in them. As a reminder, we are the only beings on the planet that can visualize a future, at least from a human perspective, and the loss of that vision can send shockwaves of helplessness. Under these circumstances, hope for the future turns into helplessness about not having a future.

Loss of Possibilities

In a more phenomenological expression of counseling and therapy, creating possibilities for clients seems an attempt to counteract the loss of possibilities that can be experienced when going through a hopeless period. However, it takes less counseling skill to mandate a medical model treatment plan or a counseling technique than to create numerous possibilities where hope can be actualized by the client—where ownership of hope can be within the client's intentionality and not the therapist. I believe as counselors we are in the "possibility business," not the probability business. It is not for us to hypothesize or to statistically guess what will hopefully work during therapy. By creating possibilities, we allow a true dialogue to take place where an agreement can be reached to move forward.

Loss of Meaning

One of my mentors, Viktor Frankl, used to say that "Despair = Suffering – Meaning" (2010). True hopelessness is experienced when all suffering and all possibilities have lost their meaning. In the above case study, Jim reached a point where he could not find any meaning left in his isolation and emotional pain. In some respects, his depression had turned more toward apathy. When depressed, you care too much, and we see this in Jim during the early stages of his depression. He felt ashamed for not being able to function. However, in the latter stages, he is out of possibilities and meaning where he now cares too little, which is more a sign of apathy than depression.[4] It may be in suicidal clients that apathy is a bigger problem than depression when counseling these clients (Ladd 2009).

Hopelessness

With no clear view of the future, followed by feeling helpless, and a loss of possibilities, leading to a loss of meaning, all together can systematically strip a person down to feeling hopeless. It seems that somewhere along this continuum a counselor could interject some form of hope into the experience. However, it seems hard to imagine hope being interjected through calculated decision-making most often used in a medical model. Here is where a more phenomenological counselor sees hope being interjected by making an intuitive decision or by having a moment of insight where what is said creates a sense of hope. Such an experience seems harder to imagine coming out of a medical model treatment plan.

A Pattern of Hope

Decide to Change Direction

I recall a story shared with me by a colleague that makes a point regarding hope. A client was feeling hopeless and not knowing what to do said to the therapist, "I need to do something, but I am afraid it won't be the right thing." The therapist replied, "Well do the wrong thing, but do something." Some believe that hope is wrapped up in feelings of optimism, and that certainly does not hurt. The brain is based on not being able to think of two thoughts at the same time, so a series of negative thoughts can only reinforce old negative neuropathways in the brain. Optimistic thoughts can reinforce positive neuropathways (Farran, Herth, and Popovich 1995). From an idealistic point of view, being optimistic seems to be a practice with positive consequences.

However, when one feels helpless, cannot see future possibilities, and has lost meaning in life, thinking positively may not be enough to turn around a traumatic negative experience. Realistically, something must change. Something must be tried, as in the above quote from my colleague, even if it turns out to be the wrong thing. Hope is based more on realism than idealism. When one's life is threatened by helpless, hopeless, and meaningless thoughts and feelings about the future, it may be time to change direction and seek out a different path regarding the past, present, and future.

For example, David kept struggling with his failure at pursuing the goal of being a lawyer like his father. He came to counseling feeling he let his parents and himself down. He tried three times to finish law school but found himself drifting away during the courses. He lost hope and was feeling helpless and lost, with regard to meaning in his life. Outside of his girlfriend, others around him were not helpful. They said things like, "It will be OK; not everyone needs to be a lawyer. Cheer up!" These attempts at optimism did not help. Ironically, they made him feel more helpless. Finally, his girlfriend said to him, "Let's not talk about law school. Let's talk about what you kept thinking when you drifted off in classes." David replied, "I think about being on the water. It is one of the few places where I feel comfortable." She said, "Why not do something on the water?" His answer was a simple, "OK, I will consider it."

Gathering Energy

At that moment in this example, David does not know whether doing something on the water is the right thing to do or the wrong thing to do, but it is something to do. Making the decision to change direction towards one's future may be more important regarding hope than whether it is the correct change or the best direction. A person can always change again. However, in the phenomenon of hope, it allows a person to gather new energy to help fill that void left by the energy exhausted from an experience that eventually lost purpose and meaning. Lack of energy promotes hopelessness. Gathering new energy does the opposite.

Hypothetically speaking, let us finish the story of David by assuming he becomes involved in the maritime industry and becomes a captain of a small salvage operation. Hope is now restored. Or, he realizes being on the water is not for him, but he changes direction again and gathers energy around public speaking and becomes a radio disc jockey. Hope is not necessarily based on what you may want to become. It holds truth to power in whether you are flexible enough to change direction and gather energy in something that energizes your future.

Transfer Energy

Being able to transfer energy from a hopeless future to a future filled with new energy is an experience that can reinforce a sense of resilience (Larsen and Stege 2012). The client realizes that he or she is not stuck in a circumstance where life cannot change. What it means from a therapeutic perspective is that a client can collaborate with a therapist on numerous possibilities for change. Many clients who seem to lose hope base it on not being able to see other possibilities for their future. Phenomenologically oriented counselors base a portion of their expertise on having a dialogue with clients to create new future possibilities. Deciding to change direction, and gather energy, places a client in a position to transfer energy into a new direction that offers the possibility of a more hopeful outlook on life.

Make It Meaningful

If one can change direction and gather energy around hope for the future, and one successfully transfers that energy, then one can sustain hope by making it meaningful. Finding meaning in a new direction in life may be one of the major reasons to seek therapy. Even if a client goes to a more medical model talk therapist and the goal of therapy is to reduce, for example, symptoms of anxiety. The client may feel more in control if symptoms are reduced through some form of counseling technique or a type of psychotropic medication. However, finding meaning through a change in personal direction, such as by gathering energy and transferring it into hope for the future, helps growth and change in the whole person. For example, John deals with his anxiety in therapy by taking Ativan and practicing cognitive/behavioral therapy. He feels more in control while he continues using both methods to face his anxiety. One day he is hit with a serious trauma where he realizes his Ativan and cognitive/behavioral skills do not work. Over time, he begins to lose hope in how to deal with anxiety, or he goes back to his mental health professional for more Ativan and more counseling techniques.

Here is the same example of John dealing with his anxiety but from a whole person perspective. John deals with his anxiety in therapy by having a meaningful dialogue with his therapist and deciding to change direction in his future. He feels more in control as he gathers energy to make this change and begins to feel more resilient when he transfers this energy into some meaningful view of a new future. One day he is hit with a serious trauma where he realizes his meaningful view of the future has lost its meaning. John realizes that he needs to make a change, so he gathers energy on his own, or by talking to a therapist, and begins to transfer that energy into a new, but different, view of his future. He has become flexible enough to deal with his anxiety when either he changes or the type of trauma changes. In either case, meaning for a new future is possible. (As a footnote, John can still go back to his mental health professional for more Ativan and more counseling techniques, but the primary difference is that John is dealing with more than symptoms. His new direction offers hope for the future through his personal ability to make change.)

Gain Flexibility

By describing hope as a practical phenomenon, it may help clients obtain hope. From deciding to gathering energy for change and transferring that energy into something meaningful, allows clients to practice a process that ends in flexibility—flexibility to decide the importance of change whenever a client begins to feel hopeless. The more a client is flexible with change, the more the client can make the decision to change. By going through the phenomenon of hope, through meaningful repetition, one is saying, "I am resilient enough to change direction if or when I begin feeling hopeless." One does not come to this point, for example, in therapy because he or she has successfully dealt with symptoms, but because she or he has successfully dealt with personal problems as a whole person.

From a neurological perspective, flexibility becomes vitally important. Negative neuropathways that have addictively embedded themselves in the minds of clients are partially responsible for problems surrounding "mental illness." From my subjective judgment, it is difficult to alter these negative neuropathways without the flexibility offered through finding a meaningful future based on hope. The mind being determined through the embodied brain, interpersonal interaction, and energy and organization happening all at once may be at the foundation of hope where attunement, insight, and intuition help in the gathering of energy. It is where meaning is found in transferring that energy into something with a purpose and having the flexibility both neurologically and phenomenologically to shift one's intentionality when old thoughts of the future have dried up.

DISCUSSION

I have observed hope in client's eyes when they have transferred energy into a meaningful future. It is not a fear of the future but confidence that they now have a future. How much of mental illness is based on not believing you have an acceptable future? Beyond the neuroscience and beyond the psychopharmacology, lies a world of experiences that have meaning for clients.

When hope enters their eyes, they are viewing their experiences as a whole person. Not only do their symptoms seem different but they as a person seem different. In some respects, it becomes difficult to capture the phenomenon of hope in therapy, or even in a chapter of a book. However, let it be said that hope is a fundamental part of the healing process when counseling mental health clients. It is one of those nuances that can be overlooked in a strictly linear, medical model approach to counseling clients. Hope seems to open the door to endless possibilities in counseling for the client and notably for the counselor. It is based on a collection of nuances not obvious to an unskilled observer. Helping a client regain hope should be a part of the skills we learn when practicing talk therapy. With hope emerges possibilities, and that is at the heart of why one practices the art of talk therapy.

One of the challenges in helping clients feel hopeful goes beyond practicing counseling skills and prescribing psychotropic drugs designed to reduce patient symptoms. Practically, using all the nuances found in hopefulness, may call for more phenomenologically based skills. Intuition, insight, attunement, empathy, and all being used through meaningful dialogue may influence the phenomenon of hope to emerge. However, these skills do not reveal a counselor's expertise but more his or her humanity.

I once hired a therapist to work in a mental health clinic on a Native American reservation. There was great promise in his expertise. Putting it honestly, even though I had numerous years of practice, he clearly knew more about counseling techniques than I could wish to know. His expertise was very humbling. However, after a few months, we as a team decided to let him go because no one wanted to go to him for counseling. As a technician he was exemplary, but as a person, he could not seriously connect with clients. He blamed it on their incompetence rather than his lack of empathy. In all fairness, there are medical model-oriented counselors who have little trouble connecting with clients and find ways to offer hope. However, from a more phenomenological viewpoint, hope is a mandatory ingredient in creating possibilities for client growth and change.

NOTES

1. The philosophy of Maurice Merleau-Ponty deepens our understanding of the rehabilitation process. The experience of chronic pain ruptures the natural connection between body and world and how the rehabilitation process can be understood as the reinsertion of the body into the flow of experience, where the body "disappears" into its natural silence to allow the world to unfold once again. The experience of chronic pain places the painful body in focus, resulting in a diminished articulation of both self and world. Persons with illness suffer not only from the physical aspects of pain and discomfort but also from a loss of identity where one feels alienated and detached from things that used to give meaning to one's life. Bullington, Jennifer. 2009. "Embodiment of Chronic Pain: Implications for Rehabilitation Practice." *Health Care Annals* 17 no. 2 (June): 100–9.

2. Rollo May presented the concept of intentionality as a client characteristic that is essential for successful therapy, and in doing so, he described intentionality as a person's inner "structure which gives meaning to experience" (p. 223). May, Rollo. 1969. *Love & Will*. New York, NY: Norton.

3. Another important aspect of counselor intentionality is the ability to seek alternative solutions and choose from an array of strategies in helping people make decisions and solve problems. In sum, the intentional counselor is one who learns many helping strategies, continues to accumulate knowledge of human development and related critical issues, and offers clients a relationship in which all possibilities can be explored, examined, and evaluated. Schmidt, John. 1994. "Counselor Intentionality and Effective Helping." *ERIC Digest*, April, EDO-CG-94-05, *https://pdfs.semanticscholar.org/b86b/633b8ec6ac46a734be2848db4495e6fa8256.pdf.*

4. Guilt is a phenomenon of the past while anxiety is a phenomenon of the future. To deal with the future when feeling anxious may require a sense of hope in helping to control one's behavior. People with apathetic feelings can compulsively create additional trauma. Apathy can cause a loss of hope and withdrawal into suicide. Ladd, Peter D. 2009. *Emotional Addictions: A Reference Book for Mental Health and Addictions Counselors.* Lanham, MD: University Press of America.

Chapter Twelve

The Talk Therapy Revolution

The twenty-first century is filled with surprises regarding talk therapy. The previous chapters point out ideological differences between a medical model compared to a more phenomenological or experiential model. Looking closely at these models, it would make sense in a century based on information and communication that a reasonable combination is possible, especially since a more phenomenological model is dialogue-centered. However, when checking that assumption in detail, neither model dominates the mental health culture, though to many the medical model appears to be the dominant model. In the actual practice of talk therapy, that assumption does not hold true. When considering the overall culture of the mental health industry, it becomes obvious, to me, that the culture moves on a more economic model rather than one based on ideology.

In my numerous discussions with talk therapists, psychologists, and psychiatrists, there are a growing number of professionals who sheepishly admit that a business model is the overriding power broker when it applies to mental health practice. Insurance companies, big pharma, and managed care facilities work from a business model where order and efficiency prevail and cost-effectiveness is the guiding force behind either ideology. From my perspective trying to revolutionize talk therapy by confronting the economics involved seems, unfortunately, the most accessible inroad. So, with a pinch of cynicism, if the client's human experience in talk therapy has any chance of being offered as a viable practice in the mental health profession, then considering the business of mental health, at this point, becomes a consideration. Furthermore, medical model practices have integrated successfully into the world of business, so it appears that experiential talk therapy has little choice but to do the same. It appears that economics is the ideological back road to a talk therapy revolution. The following are my thoughts about advocating for an experiential model being as cost-effective as a medical model and, in some cases, more cost-effective.

BUSINESS MODEL

- Both models have had an impact on mental health practice; however, I am proposing that the model that most affects the mental health industry in current society is neither of these models. My belief is that a business model now dominates the mental health industry. It appears that finances have outweighed ideology. Furthermore, one cannot assume that a medical model is more financially effective than a phenomenological model even though it appears that way, based on a medical model's popularity.
- The business model, especially in managed care facilities, in my opinion, has now taken precedence over a medical model and a phenomenological model. From a business model, there are certain variables that must be considered if a business is to be successful: 1) a business model requires a sense of order; 2) a business model requires a level of efficiency; and 3) a business model must be cost-effective.
- In facing such a cultural shift to a more business-oriented model in mental health, it is my belief that a combination of a medical model and a phenomenological (experiential) model are more orderly, efficient, and cost-effective than keeping the models separate.

Comparing Both Models from a Business Model Perspective

The following are a series of questions that are grounded in the past chapters that try to make a comparison of these two models.

How do we balance the issues of order and efficiency when comparing these models?

A medical model is designed to be orderly but not necessarily efficient. A rule-based model will always be more orderly than a model based on experience. Gathering information incrementally from the beginning when a patient comes for mental health services is a more orderly process than asking a client to share their experiences. A prime example is when a medical model reduces a diagnosis down to a collection of symptoms within a certain set of guidelines.

However, this highly organized system is designed for patients to cope with their disorders rather than heal from them. Conversely, an experiential (phenomenological) model seems more efficient though it lacks the order found in a medical model. Creating a dialogue with clients is less orderly, but the problems being resolved go deeper and are based on healing, not coping.

Under these circumstances, a combination of both models may turn out to be more cost-effective. For example, there are certain mental health disorders such as bipolar, autism, and schizophrenia, and others that the patient, family, school, and community would be thankful for some form of symptoms reduction and symptoms maintenance. A medical model may seem more appropriate for these disorders. However, a follow-up for the patient, family, school, and community as to what this means for all those involved, could be available for future views on a person's life in dealing with these types of disorders. For example, a more phenomenological method could be used to help the experience of the family regarding the impact of bipolar disorder on one of its members.

How do you compare a medical model culture and an experiential model culture for patients/clients?

In the medical model culture, there is an emphasis on accountability. A file is made for a patient that includes a diagnosis, treatment plan, assessments, family history, and progress notes. Much of this information, if practiced in an orderly fashion, makes the talk therapist accountable to the organizational guidelines and insurance companies. There is a need for proof that you are being accountable to the mental health profession.

The emphasis in an experiential model is on ability. Proof that you can establish a therapeutic alliance, stay attuned to the client, make insightful suggestions for solving of problems, and practice empathy so clients are empowered to help themselves. This becomes a more efficient way of making changes that may last longer than in symptoms reduction. Finding meaning in one's experiences seems to have a longer shelf life. Under these circumstances, a combination of both models may turn out to be more cost-effective.

How do you balance both models for the client/patient?

Simply put, a medical model follows closely with the same model as used with physically ill patients. You must prove to the patient that you know how to diagnose their problems and come up with a treatment plan to resolve these problems. The more orderly this is performed, the more competent the professionals appear to the patients. A medical model may be more appropriate for those disorders where some form of neurological and physiological crisis exists. From an experiential model, competence is derived from showing proof that you know how to create a dialogue and work with the client to let the treatment plan emerge. This appears a more efficient method for getting to problems where clients are motivated to make changes in their way of life. Under these circumstances, a medical model, a phenomenological model, or a combination of both models may turn out to be more cost-effective.

How do you balance knowledge and wisdom in both cultures for the patient/client?

In a medical model, the emphasis is on creating an orderly block of knowledge. Fundamentally, it is proof that you understand a patient's problems by making calculated decisions based on probability. Such a model may make more sense in crisis situations where stabilizing the patient is of great concern. In an experiential model, the emphasis is on wisdom, which turns out to be a more efficient method for growth and change. Proof that you can immerse yourself in a client's problems until you both intuitively know what to do based on emergent possibilities. This model puts more emphasis on the wisdom of the client, where empowerment issues can be beneficial for future meaning in the client's life. Under these circumstances, an understanding of what is more appropriate for the patient/client should be assessed where a choice of models is being offered to the patient/client, and possibly his or her families. Giving a choice between these two models may turn out to be more cost-effective.

How does one balance a medical model based on crisis intervention with an experiential healing model?

A medical model appears to be better suited both in order and efficiency for forms of crisis intervention. When in crisis, the major concern is safety, and through psychotropic drugs and immediate action by the mental health staff, order and efficiency are upheld. Crisis intervention may not be the major concern in a more experiential model, though empathy seems to have a successful impact when a client is in crisis. Overall, a medical model seems better equipped to handle crisis intervention. In this case, it appears that a medical model is more cost-effective.

How do you balance a medical model based on coping with an experiential model based on healing?

A medical model in mental health is based primarily on coping with a patient's mental health problems. This is assessed on proving you can stabilize conflict, so it does not turn into another crisis. The methods used are usually an orderly set of procedures to help patients cope. However, without some form of growth and change, patients can cope without understanding the meaning-making experiences in their lives. An experiential model appears more efficient based on the goal to help clients grow and change. A two-step process beginning with a medical model that finishes with a phenomenological model may be more cost-effective.

How do you balance psychotropic drugs with both a medical and experiential model?

In a medical model, it may be more orderly to use these drugs from the beginning to stabilize a mental health crisis. However, it may be more efficient to use drugs as a secondary approach during experiential healing. Drugs seem more efficient when used to avoid crisis and in dealing with chronic mental health problems. It seems psychotropic drugs in a more experiential model should be decided in a dialogue between client and therapist as to how long and to what degree they are necessary. A two-step process beginning with a medical model that finishes with a phenomenological model may be more cost-effective. Much as in the treatment of diabetes, taking insulin while sitting on the couch and eating jelly donuts does not holistically address the problem. In long-term care for such experiences as schizophrenia, bipolar, or possibly post-traumatic stress disorder and others, a combination of a medical and experiential models make sense.

How do you balance mental health techniques with both a medical model and an experiential model?

When mental health techniques are chosen by an expert or experts in a medical model before starting therapy or shortly thereafter, neither order nor efficiency seem to be most effective during the time one is using these techniques. Nor are these techniques more orderly or efficient when used as interventions to relieve patient symptoms. It makes more sense to use techniques as a form of education after the establishment of a therapeutic alliance. Techniques should develop out of the dialogue between therapist and client. The use of techniques at this stage seems to be more orderly and efficient.

What is the balance of power between the professional and the client/patient?

The medical model has emerged from a twenty-first-century rule-based model that is primarily organized around compliance. A more experiential model is based on twenty-first-century problem-solving model where clients are invited to problem solve with the therapist. This model is not based on compliance but on empowerment. It allows the client to be the unrecognized expert in the therapy process. What is presented during therapy is more orderly in the sense that it appears in therapy to both client and counselors and has meaning that helps order the client's life. The idea that a pharmaceutically based medical model is going to give up power in the healthcare field seems highly unlikely. However, it is more cost-effective at least for the patient/client to be empowered in some way while going through this process.

How do you balance the diagnosis between the professional and the client/ patient?

In a medical model of diagnosis, the patient is the problem. A diagnosis is presented to other experts that clarifies the disorders of the patient, and where they can label the patient for insurance, pharmaceutical, and counseling technique purposes. This is an orderly approach for diagnosing a patient. In an experiential model, the experience is the problem. Experiences emerge through dialogue that clarifies their psychological patterns and where they can apply personal meaning to these patterns. This is a more efficient way to diagnose a client based on the client finding meaning in acceptance of the pattern being presented in therapy. Under these circumstances, a medical model form of diagnosis makes sense for the "business" of mental health practice, but a more experiential model makes sense to help clients understand the pattern he or she is going through. A combination of both models may turn out to be more cost-effective.

Summary

Though the opinions in these questions are primarily based on anecdotal perceptions and over twenty-five years of repeatedly seeing results, it is my belief that there are essential elements of both phenomenological and medical model cultures that can be combined. Such a combination could result in a more accurate and cost-effective cultural shift that accounts for both medical and phenomenological beliefs and behaviors. Such a shift would not only benefit the "business" of mental health but also benefit a more well-rounded service to the patients/clients. The question of whether medical model and phenomenologically oriented professionals are willing to discuss and possibly change present mental health culture is anyone's guess. However, I believe the time is right for a talk therapy revolution by making changes in the culture of the mental health profession.

THE MENTAL HEALTH REVOLUTION: FINAL THOUGHTS

In phenomenology, it is important to view phenomena from multiple angles, and regarding mental health, looking at different angles may also be a relevant perspective. Presented in this book are two different approaches to mental health talk therapy. I have tried to critically think through both a phenomenological and a medical model approach to talking with patients/

clients. Although, there may stand out some obvious biases on my part, but overall, these models speak for themselves.

Culture plays a significant role in talk therapy practice, and the culture points to a more scientific methodology in working with people. For the most part, the medical model is built on a culture where finding the answers to mental health problems is a major goal, and if not the answers, then an attempt at probability when someone says they are depressed or anxious.

The other model, the phenomenological model, falls on a more humanistic approach to mental health. It also wants to find answers to mental health problems as a medical model, but the focus is on the client by acknowledging their unique experiences and the meanings behind them. Also, phenomenology is not looking for mental disorders embodied in the patient but is looking for possibilities to redirect one's pain into a different type of experience and a different potential future. Therefore, the client's experience becomes the problem, not a problem within the client.

So where do these models meet with the hope of minimizing pain for mental health patients/clients while maximizing benefits for mental health culture? It may mean for the more phenomenologically oriented talk therapist that trying to fit into a business model is a culturally important thing to do. This is the present-day culture in mental health and results coming from this culture offer hope for those suffering from mental health problems. However, one cannot assume that we have a dichotomy on our hands, where choosing one approach over the other will solve this cultural reality. From a present-day neuroscientific perspective, there is no reason to horde mental health culture strictly from a natural scientific perspective.

In this book, the hope is that some of the phenomenological themes presented show a possible connection between neuroscience and phenomenology, especially the experiences of clients. A medical model reaches clients in a more foundational way. Phenomenology builds on that foundation to save the unique humanity of those seeking talk therapy. Both seem important, especially for clients. This is not a predicament in the mental health industry but a problem. For the medical model to consider at least one other angle in the pursuit of mentally helping people, it does not seem out of reach. It begs the question, "Are we going to pursue the best possible mental health practice for our patients/clients, or are we going to pursue basically what is most cost-effective from a business model perspective while dominating the culture of mental health?"

If the pursuit of mental health has already transformed itself into a rigid, tightly run business, then we have already answered that question. However, if the true nature of our pursuit for helping people is ideological, then neuroscience has opened the door for a medical model and a phenomenological model to work together. Neuroscience is the common ground between the two ideologies. Neurological research has dispelled the notion that phenomenology is not scientific enough to be taken seriously, and that a medical model should unconditionally ignore the patient's experience.

It turns out that selfless acts, hope, momentum, intuition, empathy, insight, and others have a neurological importance in the field of mental health. Instead of ignoring such phenomena as not scientific enough for the culture of mental health, let us make the effort to change the culture so that these phenomenological themes have importance in the everyday practice of mental health. Join the neuroscientists and the clients in accepting their value and make room for them in mental health programs.

Finally, thousands of years ago, Homo sapiens began to talk to each other. Most likely communication was focused around survival. Nevertheless, personal communication continued through the ages where eventually different points of view were discussed and different experiences were shared. It was in the dialogue between people where we slowly molded ourselves into human beings. One could say there was a talking evolution of ideas, experiences, and points of view that got us to where we are today. However, where are we today? How do we talk to each other? What do we say that still helps in our survival? Gossip, hyperbole, verbal bullying, lies, and "fake news"—even social media—all appear more prevalent while face-to-face dialogue becomes harder to find. (Is social media bringing us closer together or creating more isolation?)

On a smaller scale, this also becomes problematic in the field of mental health. Healthy dialogue is being threatened emotionally and psychologically by some of the methods used in talk therapy. There is nothing wrong with finding mental health experts who will guide us. However, it should not be at the expense of meaningful dialogue where successful outcomes depend on both client and expert. This book was originally conceived around that thought. The presentation of neuroscience and phenomenology hopefully alludes to the importance of dialogue between human beings as a fundamental foundation in our society and in the field of mental health. In that regard, the previous pages hopefully will remind mental health professionals that bonding together through meaningful dialogue is a part of our social makeup and possibly our survival.

Glossary

Amygdala: a roughly almond-shaped mass of gray matter inside each cerebral hemisphere, involved with the experiencing of emotions.

The *anterior cingulate cortex*: is responsible for many psychological and physiological functions. It regulates blood pressure and the heart rate. Its psychological functions include decision making and evaluation processes, emotional regulation, preparation for tasks, error detection, and executive functions.

Autonomic Nervous System: the part of the nervous system responsible for control of the bodily functions not consciously directed, such as breathing, the heartbeat, and digestive processes.

Basal Ganglia: a group of structures linked to the thalamus in the base of the brain and involved in coordination of movement.

Diencephalon: the caudal (posterior) part of the forebrain, containing the epithalamus, thalamus, hypothalamus, and ventral thalamus and the third ventricle.

Dopamine: A monoamine neurotransmitter that is formed during the synthesis of norepinephrine and is essential to the normal functioning of the central nervous system. A reduction of dopamine in the brain is associated with the development of Parkinson's disease.

Dorsomedial Prefrontal Cortex: is a section of the prefrontal cortex (PFC). It is involved in creating a sense of the self. This sense of self that the dorsomedial prefrontal cortex is involved in is what referred to as "me-ness." It is also involved in what is called "Theory of mind," or considering the mental states of others. Brain activity in the dorsomedial prefrontal cortex has been shown to be significant in altruism.

Endorphins: any of a group of hormones secreted within the brain and nervous system and having different physiological functions. They are peptides that activate the body's opiate receptors, causing an analgesic effect.

Executive Functions: are a set of processes that all have to do with managing oneself and one's resources to achieve a goal. It is an umbrella term for the neurologically-based skills involving mental control and self-regulation.

The *GABA*: receptors are a class of receptors that respond to the neurotransmitter gamma-aminobutyric acid (GABA), the chief inhibitory compound in the mature vertebrate central nervous system.

Hippocampus: the elongated ridges on the floor of each lateral ventricle of the brain, thought to be the center of emotion, memory, and the autonomic nervous system.

Hypothalamus: a region of the forebrain below the thalamus that coordinates both the autonomic nervous system and the activity of the pituitary, controlling body temperature, thirst, hunger, and other homeostatic systems, and involved in sleep and emotional activity.

The *hypothalamic–pituitary–adrenal axis (HPA axis or HTPA axis)*: is a complex set of direct influences and feedback interactions among three components: the hypothalamus, the pituitary gland (a pea-shaped structure located below the thalamus), and the adrenal (also called "suprarenal") glands (small, conical organs on top of the kidneys). These organs and their interactions constitute the HPA axis, a major neuroendocrine system that controls reactions to stress and regulates many body processes, including digestion, the immune system, mood and emotions, sexuality, and energy storage and expenditure.

Insula: The insulae are believed to be involved in consciousness and play a role in diverse functions usually linked to emotion or the regulation of the body's homeostasis. These functions include compassion and empathy, perception, motor control, self-awareness, cognitive functioning, and interpersonal experience.

The *insular cortex*: particularly its most anterior portion, is considered a limbic-related cortex. In terms of function, the insula is believed to process convergent information to produce an emotionally relevant context for sensory experience.

Integrated Mind: The most immediately shocking element of this definition is that our mind extends beyond our physical selves. In other words, our mind is not simply our perception of experiences, but those experiences themselves.

The primary structures within the *limbic system*: include the amygdala, hippocampus, thalamus, hypothalamus, basal ganglia, and cingulate gyrus. The amygdala is the emotion center of the brain, while the hippocampus plays an essential role in the formation of new memories about past experiences.

The *locus coeruleus*: also spelled locus caeruleus or locus ceruleus is a nucleus in the pons of the brainstem involved with physiological responses to stress and panic.

A *mirror neuron*, or *cubelli neuron*: is a neuron that fires both when an animal acts and when the animal observes the same action performed by another. Thus, the neuron "mirrors" the behavior of the other, as though the observer were itself acting. Such neurons have been directly observed in primate species.

Neuroplasticity: the ability of the brain to form and reorganize synaptic connections, especially in response to learning or experience or following injury.

Neurogenesis: the growth and development of nervous tissue.

Parasympathetic Nervous System: The part of the involuntary nervous system that serves to slow the heart rate, increase intestinal and glandular activity, and relax the sphincter muscles. The parasympathetic nervous system, together with the sympathetic nervous system, constitutes the autonomic nervous system.

Prefrontal Cortex: the gray matter of the anterior part of the frontal lobe that is highly developed in humans and plays a role in the regulation of complex cognitive, emotional, and behavioral functioning.

The *supra marginal gyrus*: is part of the somatosensory association cortex, which interprets tactile sensory data and is involved in perception of space and limbs location. It is also involved in identifying postures and gestures of other people, and is thus a part of the mirror neuron system.

Functionally, the *striatum*: coordinates multiple aspects of cognition, including motor- and action-planning, decision-making, motivation, reinforcement, and reward perception

The *superior temporal gyrus* contains the primary auditory cortex, which is responsible for processing sounds. . . . The superior temporal gyrus also includes the Wernicke's area, which (in most people) is located, in the left hemisphere. It is the major area involved in the comprehension of language.

Sympathetic Nervous System: the part of the autonomic nervous system that contains chiefly adrenergic fibers and tends to depress secretion, decrease the tone and contractility of smooth muscle, and increase heart rate—compare parasympathetic nervous system.

Vagus Nerve: A nerve that supplies nerve fibers to the pharynx (throat), larynx (voice box), trachea (windpipe), lungs, heart, esophagus, and intestinal tract, as far as the transverse portion of the colon.

Ventromedial Prefrontal Cortex (vmPFC): is a part of the prefrontal cortex in the mammalian brain. The ventral medial prefrontal cortex is located, in the frontal lobe at the bottom of the cerebral hemispheres and is implicated in the processing of risk and fear.

References

Abdou, Adham, S. Higashiguchi, Kim Horie, and Hatucui Yokogoshi. 2006. "Relaxation and Immunity Enhancement Effects of Gamma-Aminobutyric Acid (GABA) Administration in Humans." *Biofactors* 26 no. 3 (April): 201–8.

Alexander, John. 2017. *The Journey Begins with 1,000 Miles: Thriving with Parkinson's Disease Through Hope, Optimism, and Perseverance*. New York, NY: Positively Powered Publications.

Aldao, Amelia. 2014. "Emotional Regulation: What Is It and Why Does It Matter." *Psychology Today*, August 29, 2017.

Allen, Summer, and Jill Suttie. 2015. "How the Brain Makes Us Generous." *Greater Good Science Center: Berkley California*, January 2015. https://greatergood.berkeley.edu/.

Adolphs, Richard, David Tranel, Hanna Damasio, and Antonio Damasio. 1995. "Fear and the Human Amygdala." The Journal of Neuroscience 15 (9): 5879–91.

American Psychiatric Association. 2013. *Diagnostic and Statistical Manual-5*. Washington, DC: American Psychological Association.

Barsky, Allan. 2017. "*DSM-5* and the Ethics of Diagnosis." *The New Social Worker Magazine* (April): 43.

Bavol'ár, Jozef and Ol'ga Orosová. 2015. "Decision Making Styles and their Associations with Decision-Making Competencies and Mental Health." *Judgment and Decision Making* 10 no.1 (January): 115–122.

Bechara, Antione, Hanna Damasio, Antonio Damasio, and Gregory Lee. 1999. "Different Contributions of the Human Amygdala and the Ventromedial Prefrontal Cortex to Decision-Making." *Journal of Neuroscience* 19 no. 13 (August): 5473–81.

Bedi, Robinder, Michael Davis and Meris Williams. 2005. "Critical Incidents in the Formation of the Therapeutic Alliance from the Client's Perspective." *Psychotherapy Theory Research Practice Training.* 42 no. 3 (Fall): 311–323.

Bender, Donna S. 2005. "Therapeutic Alliance," in *The American Psychiatric Publishing Textbook of Personality Disorders*. Edited by Andrew Oldham, Ed. Skodol, and Donna S. Bender. Washington, DC: American Psychiatric Publishing, Inc., 405–20.

Benedetti, Fabrizio, Elisa Carlino, and Antonella Pollo. 2011. "How Placebo Change the Patient's Brain." *Neuropsychopharmacology* 36 no.1 (January): 339–54.

Bennington, Vanessa. 2010. "The Ups and Downs of Cortisol: What You Need to Know." *Textbook of Functional Medicine.* Gig Harbor, WA: Institute of Functional Medicine. https://breakingmuscle.com/fitness/the-ups-and-downs-of-cortisol-what-you-need-to-know

Bergland, Christopher. 2012. "The Neurochemicals of Happiness." *Psychology Today,* November 29, 2012.

Berlucchi, Giovani and Salvitore Aglioti. 1997. "The Body in the Brain: Neural Bases of Corporeal Awareness." *Trends in Neuroscience* 20 (1997): 560–4.

Bien, Thomas. 2006. *Mindful Therapy*. Somerville, MA: Wisdom Publications.

Blake, Holly. 2017. "What Happens to Your Body When You're Stressed?" *Neuroscience News*, August 9, 2017.

Bocanegra, B. R. and R. Zeelenberg. 2011. "Emotional Cues Enhance the Attentional Effects on Spatial and Temporal Resolution." Psychonomic Bulletin & Review 18 no.6 (September): 1071–76. DOI 10.3758/s13423-011-0156-z.

Bowden, Edward, Mark Jung-Beeman, Jessica Fleck, and John Kounios. 2005. "New Approaches to Demystifying Insight." *Trends in Cognitive Science* 9 no.7 (July): 322–28.

Bozarth, Jerold D. 2009. "Rogerian Empathy in an Organismic Theory: A Way of Being," In *Social Neuroscience of Empathy.* Edited by Jean Decety and William Ickes. Cambridge, MA: MIT Press, 101–12.

Breuning, Lorreta G. 2016. *The Science of Positivity: Stop Negative Thought Patterns by Changing Your Brain Chemistry.* Avon, MA: Adams Media.

Brown, Richard. 2013. *Consciousness Inside and Out: Phenomenology, Neuroscience, and the Nature of Experience.* New York, NY: Springer Science.

Buber, Martin. 2014. *Between Man & Man.* Eastford, CT: Martino Fine Books.

Bullington, Jennifer. 2009. "Embodiment of Chronic Pain: Implications for Rehabilitation Practice." *Health Care Annals* 17 no. 2 (June): 100–9. doi 10.1007/s10728-008-0109-5.

Bush, George, Phan Luu, and Michael Posner. 2000. "Cognitive and Emotional Influences in Anterior Cingulate Cortex Trends." *Trends in Cognitive Science* 4, no. 6 (June): 215–22.

Cacioppo, John T, Gary G. Berntson, and Howard C. Nusbaum. 2008. "Neuroimaging as a New Tool in the Toolbox of Psychological Science." Current Directions in Psychological Science 17, no. 2 (April): 62–7.

Carlson, Linda. 2015. "The Placebo Effect & the Healing Relationship: Somatic Perspectives." Accessed December 2015. https://relationalimplicit.com/carlson.

Carpenter, Siri. 2012. "That Gut Feeling." *American Psychological Association* 43 no.8 (September): 50.

Castrén, Edward. 2005. "Is Mood Chemistry?" *Nature Reviews Neuroscience* 6 no. 3 (March): 241–6.

Cavanagh, Sarah R. 2013. "Your Brain on Friendship." *Psychology Today*, May 30, 2013.

Chamodraka, Martha, Marilyn Fitzpatrick, and Jennifer Janzen. 2017. "Hope as Empowerment Model: A Client-Based Perspective on the Development of Hope." *The Journal of Positive Psychology* 12 no. 3 (Spring): 232–45.

Colaizzi, Paul F. 1978. "Psychological Research as the Phenomenologist Views It." In *Existential-Phenomenological Alternatives for Psychology.* Edited by Ronald Valle and Mark King. Oxford, UK: Oxford University Press, 6.

Craig, Bud A. D. 2009. "Emotional Moments Across Time: A Possible Neural Basis for Time Perception in the Anterior Insula." *Philosophical Transactions of the Royal Society: Biological Sciences* 364 no. 1525 (July): 1933–42. http://doi.org/10.1098/rstb.2009.0008.

Craig, Bud A. D. 2009. "How Do You Feel—Now? The Anterior Insula and Human Awareness." Nature Reviews Neuroscience 10 no. 1 (January): 59–70. PMID: 19096369

Cronin, Elisabeth, Bethany L. Brand, and Jonathan F. Mattanah. 2014. "The Impact of the Therapeutic Alliance on Treatment Outcome in Patients with Dissociative Disorders." *European Journal of Psychotraumatology* 5 no.10 (March): 3402.

Damasio, Antonio. 2005. *Descartes' Error: Emotion, Reason, and the Human Brain.* New York, NY: Penguin Books.

Damasio, Antonio. 2000. *The Feeling of What Happens: Body and Emotion in the Making of Consciousness*. New York, NY: Mariner Books.

Dane, Eric, Kevin W. Rockmann, and Michael G. Pratt. 2012. "When Should I Trust My Gut? Linking Domain Expertise to Intuitive Decision-Making Effectiveness," *Organizational Behavior and Human Decision Processes* 119 no. 2 (November): 187–94.

Daw, Nathaniel, and Philippe Tobler. 2014. "Value Learning through Reinforcement: The Basics of Dopamine and Reinforcement Learning." Chap. 15, 283–94. *Neuroeconomics.* Cambridge, MA: Academic Press.

DeAngelis, Tori. 2008. "The Two Faces of Oxytocin: Why Does the 'Tend and Befriend' Hormone Come Into Play at the Best and Worst of Times?" *Science Watch* 39, no. 2 (February): 30.

Decety, Jean. 2010. "The Neurodevelopment of Empathy in Humans." *Developmental Neuroscience* 32 no. 4 (December): 257–67.

De Groot, Jasper, Monique Smeets, and Gün Semin. 2015. "Rapid Stress System Drives Chemical Transfer of Fear from Sender to Receiver." *PLOS ONE* 10, no. 2 (February): e0118211. https://doi.org/10.1371/journal.pone.0118211.

Dehaene, Stanislas. 2014. *Consciousness and the Brain: Deciphering How the Brain Codes Our Thoughts*. New York, NY: Penguin Group.

Duckworth, Ken. 2015. "Science Meets the Human Experience: Integrating the Medical Model and Recovery Model." *National Alliance on Mental Illness* (April 10): 35–45.

Duggan, Jamie M, Jessica R. Toste, and Nancy L. Heath. 2013. "An Examination of the Relationship between Body Image Factors and Non-Suicidal Self-Injury in Young Adults: The Mediating Influence of Emotion Dysregulation." *Psychiatry Research* 206, Nos. 2–3 (April): 256–64.

Ecker, Bruce, Robin Ticic, and Laurel Hulley. 2012. *Unlocking the Emotional Brain: Eliminating Symptoms at Their Roots Using Memory Reconsolidation.* London, UK: Routledge.

Egan, Danielle. 2017. "Person-Centered Diagnosis and Treatment in Mental Health: A Model for Empowering Clients." *New York State Psychological Association Presentation* (June 2): 2.

Eldar, Eran, Robb Rutledge, Raymond Dolan, and Yael Niv. 2015. "Mood as Representation of Momentum." *Trends in Cognitive Sciences* 20, no. 1 (January): 15–24.

Erksine, Richard G. 1998. "Attunement and Involvement: Therapeutic Responses to Relational Needs." *International Journal of Psychotherapy* 3 no. 3 (November): 235–44.

Fall, Kevin, Janice Miner Holden, and Andre Marquis. 2016. *Theoretical Models of Counseling and Psychotherapy.* New York, NY: Routledge.

Farran, Carol, Kaye Herth, and Judith Popovich. 1995. *Hope and Hopelessness: Critical Clinical Constructs.* Thousand Oaks, CA: SAGE Publications.

Feather, Nicholas. 1968. " Change in Confidence Following Success or Failure as a Predictor of Subsequent Performance." *Journal of Personality and Social Psychology* 9, no. 1 (January): 38–46.

Felder, Andrew J. and Brent D. Robbins. 2016. "The Integrated Heart of Cultural and Mindfulness Meditation Practice in Existential Phenomenology and Humanistic Psychotherapy." *The Humanistic Psychologist* 44 no.2 (March): 105–26.

Figley, Charles R. 2002. *Treating Compassion Fatigue.* London, UK: Routledge, Psychosocial Series.

Fiora, Carlin. 2017. "Gut Almighty." *Psychology Today,* February 10, 2017. http//www.psychoilogy today.com.

Forte, Tiago. 2017. "Moods Are the Brain's Way of Creating Momentum." *Thrive Global,* June 9, 2017. https://journal.thriveglobal.com/the-psychology-behind-why-fake-it-til-you-make-it-works-in-so-many-situations-b2713bae6c2c.

Fosha, Diana, Daniel Siegel, and Marion Solomon. 2009. *The Healing Power of Emotion: Affective Neuroscience, Development & Clinical Practice.* New York, NY: W. W. Norton & Company.

Frankl, Viktor. 2014. *The Will to Meaning: Foundations and Applications of Logo therapy.* London, UK: Penguin Group.

———. 2010. *The Doctor and the Soul: From Psychotherapy to Logo Therapy*. New York, NY: Vintage Books.

———. 2009. *The Unheard Cry for Meaning: Psychotherapy and Humanism.* New York, NY: Touchstone Publishers.

———. 1973. *Psychotherapy and Existentialism: Selected Papers on Logo-therapy.* New York, NY: Pelican Books.

———. 1967. *Psychotherapy and Existentialism: Selected Papers on Logo-therapy.* New York, NY: Simon & Schuster.

Giorgi, A. 2009. *Descriptive Phenomenological Method in Psychology*. Pittsburgh, PA: Duquesne University Press.
———. 1983. “Concerning the Possibility of Phenomenological Psychological Research.” *Research Gate* 4 no. 27 (January): 129–69.
———. 1970. *Psychology as a Human Science: A Phenomenological Based Approach*. New York, NY: Harper & Row.
Gladwell, Malcolm. 2007. *Blink: The Power of Thinking without Thinking*. New York, NY: Back Bay Books.
Gonzalez, Robbie. 2011. “How Scientists Discovered the ‘Fear Center’ of the Brain.” *io9* October 12, 2011. https://io9.gizmodo.com/5848960/how-does-your-brain-process-fear/.
Grecucci, Alessandro and Remo Job. 2015. “Rethinking Reappraisal: Insights from Affective Neuroscience.” *Behavioral and Brain Science* 38 (September): e102. doi: 10.1017/S0140525X14001538.
Hansen, James T. 2016. *Meaning Systems and Mental Health Culture: Critical Perspectives on Contemporary Counseling and Psychotherapy*. Lanham, MD: Lexington Books.
Hanson, Rick. 2013. *Hardwiring Happiness: The New Brain Science of Contentment, Calm, and Confidence*. New York, NY: Harmony Publications.
Heidegger, Martin. 1996. *Being and Time*. Albany NY: New York State University of New York Press.
Hubbard, Timothy. 2015. “The Varieties of Momentum-Like Experience.” *Psychological. Bulletin* 141 no. 6 (November): 1081–119.
———. 2015. “ Forms of Momentum Across Time: Behavioral and Psychological.” *Journal of Mind & Behavior* 36 nos. 1 and 2 (Spring): 47–82.
Hunt, Carly, Jeremy Rietschel, Bradley Hatfield, and Seppo Iso-Ahola. 2013. “ A Psychophysiological Profile of Winners and Losers in Sport Competition.” *Sport, Exercise, and Performance Psychology* 2 no.3: 220–31. http://dx.doi.org/10.1037/a0031957.
Iacoboni, Marco. 2009. *Mirroring People: The Science of Empathy and How We connect with Others*. New York, NY: Picador Publications.
———. 2006. “The Mirror Neuron Revolution: Explaining What Makes Humans Social” *Scientific American,* September 10, 2006. https://www.scientificamerican.com/article/the-mirror-neuron-revolut/.
Iso-Ahola, Seppo and Charles Dotson. 2016. “Psychological Momentum—A Key to Continued Success.” *Frontiers of Psychology* 7 (August 31): 1328.
Iso-Ahola, Seppo and Ken Mobily. 1980. “Psychological Momentum: A Phenomenon and an Empirical (Unobtrusive) Validation of its Influence in a Competitive Sport Tournament.” *Psychological Reports* 46, no. 2 (January): 391–401.
Ivey, Allan and John J. Ratey. 2009. *Neuroscience and the Brain: Implications for Counseling and Therapy* (DVD Format). Accessed December 3, 2009, ASIN 1463111967.
Jacob, K. S. and V. Patel. 2014. “Classification of Mental Disorders: A Global Mental Health Perspective.” *Indian Journal of Psychological Medicin* e 383 (April):1433–5. doi: 10.1016/S0140-6736(13)62382-X.
Kabat-Zinn, Jon. 2005. *Coming to Our Senses: Healing Ourselves and the World Through Mindfulness*. London, UK: Hatchett Books.
Kays, Jill L., Robert Hurley, and Katherine H. Taber. 2012. “The Dynamic Brain: Neuroplasticity and Mental Health,” *Applied Neuropsychology* 24 no. 2 (April): 118–24.
Kounios, John and Mark Beeman. 2009. “The *Aha!* Moment: The Cognitive Neuroscience of Insight.” *Current Directions in Psychological Science* 18 no. 4 (August): 14.
Kumfor, Fiona and Sicong Tu. 2015. “Can Your Brain Really Be ‘Full’?” *The Conversation,* June 2, 2015. https://www.scientificamerican.com/article/can-your-brain-really-be-full/.
Ladd, Peter D. 2017. “Why Emotional Addictions Rob You of Feeling Fully Human: Implications for Addictions and Mental Health Counselors,” *New York State Psychological Association,* June 3, 2017.
———. 2016. “A Scar is Not a Wound: A Metaphor for Counseling.” *Counseling Today,* November 10, 2016.
———. 2013. “Knowledge vs. Wisdom in *DSM* Diagnosis: A Person-Centered Perspective,” *VISTA*: *Washington, DC: American Counseling Association* (April): Article 6.

———. 2012. "Where is Mental Health Diagnosis Heading, and Where Does It Fall Short?" *IMH Blog. Nottingham, UK: Institute of Mental Health,* October 12, 2012.

———. 2009. *Emotional Addictions: A Reference Book for Mental Health and Addictions Counselors.* Lanham, MD: University Press of America.

Ladd, Peter D. and Kyle E. Blanchfield. 2016. *Mediation, Conciliation, and Emotions: The Role of Emotional Climate in Understanding Violence and Mental Illness,* Revised Edition. Lanham, MD: Lexington Books.

Ladd, Peter D. and Ann Marie Churchill. 2012. *Person-Centered Diagnosis and Treatment in Mental Health: A Model for Empowering Clients.* London, UK: Jessica Kingsley Publishing, 1–25.

Larsen, Denise and Rachel Stege. 2012. "Client Accounts of Hope in Early Counseling Sessions: A Qualitative Study." *Journal of Counseling & Development* 90 no. 1 (January): 45–54.

Larsen, Denise, Wendy Edey, and Lenora Lemay. 2007. "Understanding the Role of Hope in Counseling: Exploring the Intentional Uses of Hope." *Counseling Psychology Quarterly* 20 no. 4 (December): 401–16.

LeDoux, Joseph and Daniel S. Pine. 2016. "Using Neuroscience to Help Understand Fear and Anxiety: A Two-System Framework." *American Journal of Psychiatry* 173, no. 11 (September): 1083–93. doi: 10.1176/appi.ajp.2016.16030353.

LeDoux, Joseph. 2012. "Rethinking the Emotional Brain." *Neuron* 73, no. 4 (February): 653–76.

Lang, Peter J., and Margret M. Bradley. 2010. "Emotion and the Motivational Brain." *Biological Psychology* 84 no.3 (June): 437–50.

Lewis, Marc. 2016. *The Biology of Disease: Why Addiction is Not a Disease.* New York, NY: Public Affairs Reprint.

Linhorst, Donald. 2006. *Empowering People with Severe Mental Illness: A Practical Guide.* Oxford, UK: Oxford University.

Littrell, Jill. 2015. *Neuroscience for Psychologists and Other Mental Health Professionals: Promoting Well-Being and Treating Mental Illness.* New York, NY: Springer Publications.

London, Scott. 2018. *The Power of Dialogue.* http://www.scottlondon.com/articles/ondialogue.html

Lopez, Shane J., Jennifer Teramoto Pedrotti, and C. R. Snyder. 2014. *Positive Psychology: The Scientific and Practical Explorations of Human Strengths.* Thousand Oaks, CA: SAGE Publications.

Lufityanto, Galang, Chris Donkin, and Joel Pearson. 2016. "Measuring Intuition: Nonconscious Emotional Information Boosts Decision Accuracy and Confidence," *Psychological Science* 27, no. 5 (April 6, 2016): 622–34. doi:10.1177/0956797616629403.

Luke, Chad. 2015. *Neuroscience for Counselors and Therapists: Integrating the Sciences of Mind and Brain.* Thousand Oaks, CA: SAGE Publications.

Marts, Arnaud C. 1966. *The Generosity of Americans: Its Source, Its Achievements.* Englewood Cliffs, NJ: Prentice-Hall.

May, Rollo. 1969. *Love & Will.* New York, NY: Norton.

McGonigal, Kelly. 2010. "Why We Need a Little Fear." *Psychology Today,* December 14, 2010. https://www.psychologytoday.com/blog/the-science-willpower/201012/why-we-need-little-fear.

McKay, Sarah. 2017. "Neuroscience Insight: How to Break Bad Habits." *The Chopra Center,* 7: 322–28.

McRae, Kateri, Supriya Misra, Adtitya Prasad, Susan Pereira, and James J. Gross. 2011. "Bottom-up and Top-down Emotion Generation: Implications for Emotion Regulation." Social Cognitive and Affective Neuroscience 7 no. 3 (February): 253–62.

Merleau-Ponty, Maurice. 2002. *Phenomenology of Perception.* London, UK: Routledge Classics.

———. 1992. *Sense and Nonsense.* Chicago, IL: Northwestern University Press.

Miller, William and Steven Rollnick. 2012. *Motivational Interviewing: Helping People Change.* New York, NY: Guilford Publications.

Miller, William R. and Steven Rollnick. 2002. Motivational Interviewing: Preparing People to Change. New York, NY: Guilford Press.

Nanda, Jyoti. 2009. "Mindfulness: A Lived Experience of Existential-Phenomenological Themes." *Existential Analysis* 20, no. 1 (January):114–31.

Norton, John. 2016. "How Einstein Did Not Discover," *Physics in Perspective* 18: 249–82.

Patoine, Brenda. 2016. "The Mindful Brain: White-Matter May Explain Behavioral Effects of Mindfulness Meditation Practices." *Dana Foundation,* May 31, 2016. http://www.dana.org/Briefing_Papers/The_Mindful_Brain/.

Rock, David. 2009. "The Neuroscience of Mindfulness." *Psychology Today,* October 11, 2009. https://www.psychologytoday.com/blog/your-brain-work/200910/the-neuroscience-mindfulness.

Roeper, John. 2013. "Dissecting the Diversity of Midbrain Dopamine Neurons." *Trends in Neuroscience* 36 no. 6 (June): 336–42.

Rogers, Carl. 2003. *Client-Centered Therapy: Its Current Practice, Implications, and Theory.* New York, NY: Robinson Publishing.

———. 1992. "The Processes of Therapy." Journal of Consulting and Clinical Psychology 60 no. 2 (April): 163–64.

———. 1980. *A Way of Being.* New York, NY: Houghton and Mifflin.

———. 1951. *Client-Centered Therapy: Its Current Practice, Implications and Theory.* Boston, MA: Houghton Mifflin.

Rosenqvist, Olof and Oskar Nordström Skans. 2015. "Confidence Enhanced Performance?: The Causal Effects of Success on Future Performance in Professional Golf Tournaments." *Journal of Economic Behavior & Organization* 117 (June): 281–95.

Rossouw, Pieter. 2013. "The End of the Medical Model? Recent Findings in Neuroscience Regarding Antidepressant Medication: Implications for Neuropsychotherapy." Neuropsychothearpy in Australia 1 (2013): 3–10.

Segerstrom, Suzanne. 2011. "The Structure and Consequences of Repetitive Thought." *Psychological Science Agenda,* (March): 34–5.

Sharot, Tali and Raymond J. Dolan. 2012. *Neuroscience a Preference and Choice: Cognitive and Neural Mechanisms.* London, UK: Academic Press.

Shpancer, Noam. 2010. "Overcoming Fear: The Only Way Out is Through." *Psychology Today,* September 10, 2010. https://www.psychologytoday.com/blog/insight-therapy/201009/overcoming-fear-the-only-way-out-is-through.

Siegel, Daniel. 2016. *Mind: A Journey to the Heart of Being Human.* New York, NY: W. W. Norton & Company.

———. 2015. *The Developing Mind.* New York, NY: The Guilford Press.

———. 2012. *Pocket Guide to Interpersonal Neurobiology: An Integrative Handbook of the Mind.* New York, NY: W. W. Norton & Company.

———. 2010. *The Mindful Brain: The Neurobiology of Well-Being.* New York, NY: W. W. Norton & Company.

———. 2010. *The Mindful Therapist: A Clinician's Guide to Mindsight and Neural Integration.* New York, NY: W. W. Norton & Company.

Simsek, Dennis. 2017. "Cortisol Levels and Anxiety: The Ultimate Guide." *The Anxiety Guy,* May 6, 2017. https://anxietyexit.com/cortisol-levels-anxiety/.

Sincero, Sahara M. 2017. "Top-Down vs. Bottom-Up Processing." *Explorable.com,* September 30, 2017. https://explorable.com/top-down-vs-bottom-up-processing.

Singleton, Oscar, et al. 2014. "Change in Brainstem Gray Matter Concentration Following a Mindfulness-Based Intervention is Correlated with Improvement in Psychological Well-Being." Frontiers in Human Neuroscience 8 no. 33 (July): 47–67.

Skjaerven, Knut. 2009. "Phenomenology: What is Intentionality?" *Barebones Communication,* February 2009.

Solomon, Marion and Daniel Siegel. 2017. *How People Change: Relationships and Neuro Plasticity in Psychotherapy.* New York, NY: W. W. Norton & Company.

Spinelli, Ernesto. 2005. *The Interpreted World. An Introduction to Phenomenological Psychology,* 2nd Edition. London: SAGE Publications.

Stahl, Bob, and Elisha Goldstein. 2010. *A Mindfulness-Based Stress Reduction Workbook.* Oakland, CA: New Harbinger Publishing.

Suzuki, Ayako. 2012. "Emotional Functions of the Insula." *Brain Nerve* 64 no.10 (October): 1103–12.

Turner, Victoria. 2016. "It Takes Effort to Be Selfish." *Medical Daily,* 2016, 111–14.

van den Berg, Jan. 1972. *A Different Existence.* Pittsburgh, PA: Duquesne University Press.

Van Gordon, William., Edo Shonin, Mark D. Griffiths, and Nirbhay N. Singh. 2015. "There is Only One Mindfulness: Why Science and Buddhism Need to Work Together." *Mindfulness* 6 no.1 (February): 49–56.

Wager, Tor et al. 2004. "Placebo-Induced Changes in fMRI in the Anticipation and Experience of Pain." *Science* 303 no. 5661 (February): 1162–67.

Waytz, Adam, Jamil Zaki, and Jason Mitchell. 2012. "Response of Dorsomedial Prefrontal Cortex Predicts Altruistic Behavior." *Journal of Neuroscience U.S. National Library of Medicine* 32 no. 22 (July): 7646–50.

Wheeler, Megan S, Diane B. Arnkoff, and Carol R. Glass. 2017. "The Neuroscience of Mindfulness: How Mindfulness Alters the Brain and Facilitates Emotion Regulation." *Mindfulness Journal* 8 (2017): 1471–87.

Whitbourne, Susan. 2015. "Our Top-Down Brains and How They Help Us Adapt to the World." *Psychology Today,* February 28, 2015. https://www.psychologytoday.com/blog/fulfillment-any-age/201502/our-top-down-brains-and-how-they-help-us-adapt-the-world.

Wilson, Ian. 2013. "Overwhelming Generosity." *British Dental Journal* 214 no. 11(Spring): 541.

Yarrow, Kielan, Peter Brown, and John W. Krakauer. 2009. "Inside the Brain of an Elite Athlete: The Neural Processes that Support High Achievement in Sports." *Nature Reviews Neuroscience* 10, no. 8 (August): 585–96.

Young, J. Scott, and Craig Cashwell. 2017. *Clinical Mental Health Counseling: Elements of Effective Practice.* Thousand Oaks, CA: SAGE Publishing.

Zaki, Jamil, Gilberto López, and Jason Mitchell. 2014. "Activity in Ventromedial Prefrontal Cortex Co-Varies with Revealed Social Preferences: Evidence for Person-Invariant Value." *Social Cognitive Affective Neuroscience* 9 no. 4 (January): 464–9.

Zimmerman, Marc 2000. Empowerment Theory. Handbook of Community Psychology. pp. 43–63.

Zubieta, Jon-Kar and Christian Stohler. 2009. "Neurobiological Mechanisms of Placebo Responses." *Annals of the New York Academy of Sciences* 1156 no.1 (March): 198–210.

Index

About the Author

Peter D. Ladd, PhD, has been a tenured faculty member at St. Lawrence University in the Graduate School of Education for over thirty-five years. He coordinates the Mental Health Counseling Program—an existential phenomenological approach to mental health counseling. Also, he has worked for thirty-eight years with St. Lawrence University's satellite graduate school program on the Akwesasne Mohawk Reservation. Over his career, Dr. Ladd worked as a graduate assistant for Viktor Frankl in the mid-1970s, and worked with Carl Rogers as a contributing author for the book *Freedom to Learn for the Eighties*, and attended Duquesne University where he studied existential phenomenology. This will be his twelfth book, all of which have had a phenomenological emphasis, with one winning a national book award. He has written numerous articles in the areas of addictions counseling, mental health counseling, relationship counseling, and conflict resolution. Dr. Ladd also works on the Akwesasne Mohawk Reservation where he established two mental health counseling centers and was the licensed clinical supervisor for the Tekanikonrahwa:kon Wholistic Health & Wellness Program, working closely with native healers from the tribe. He is presently working as a trauma consultant for the Saint Regis Mohawk Tribal Police dealing with domestic violence and post-traumatic stress disorder.

Lightning Source UK Ltd.
Milton Keynes UK
UKHW01n2212210918
329305UK00001B/30/P

9 781498 57678